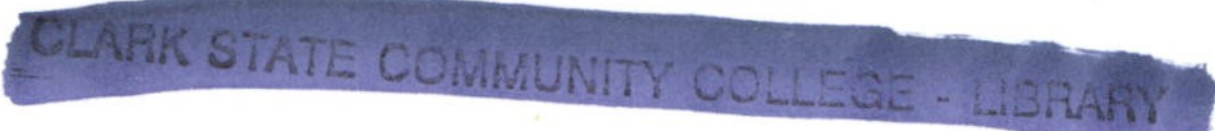

CARE of the Cancer Patient

A quick reference guide

Wesley C Finegan
MB BCh, BAO, MRCGP, MICGP, D Pall Med

and

Angela McGurk
RGN, Dip Ed

With contributions by Wilma O'Donnell and Jan Pederson

Foreword by

Dr Elizabeth Rogerson
Head of Education and Development, International Virtual Nursing School
Head, Distance Learning Centre (Nursing and Palliative Care), University of Dundee

Radcliffe Publishing
Oxford • New York

Radcliffe Publishing Ltd
18 Marcham Road
Abingdon
Oxon OX14 1AA
United Kingdom

www.radcliffe-oxford.com
Electronic catalogue and worldwide online ordering facility.

New research and clinical experience can result in changes in treatment and drug therapy. Readers of this book should therefore check the most recent product information on any drug they may prescribe to ensure they are complying with the manufacturer's recommendations concerning dosage, the method and duration of administration, and contraindications. Neither the publisher nor the authors accept liability for any injury or damage arising from this publication.

British Library Cataloguing in Publication Data

A catalogue record for this book is available from the British Library.

ISBN-10 1 84619 128 9
ISBN-13 978 1 84619 128 2

Typeset by Lapiz Digital Services, Chennai
Printed and bound by TJI Digital, Padstow, Cornwall

This book is dedicated to the memory of Alice Finegan, a loving wife, devoted mother, loyal friend to all who knew her and cancer patient, who died on 29 August 2005, aged 53 years.

Alice's last wish was that fellow cancer patients receive as good and effective care as she did herself, and that they die with the dignity and peace she knew in her last days.

WCF

In memory of my much loved 'big sis', Margaret Anne Stewart, a cancer patient, died 11 November 2006, aged 46.

AMcG

Our father, Wesley, sadly lost his own battle with cancer just days after making the final corrections to this manuscript. As his children, we were so pleased that he was able to fulfil his ambition of completing this, his third book.

CWF and SAD

Contents

Foreword vii
Preface ix
About the authors xi
Acknowledgements xii
Resource texts xiii
What standards of treatment and care can the patient reasonably expect? xiv

Part 1 Communicating with the patient
1 Basic issues in communication 2
2 Listening effectively: 'ALWAYS REACT' 6
Jan Pederson
3 Breaking bad news 15
4 The angry patient 19
5 Collusion 23
6 Confidentiality 26
7 Denial 28
8 Distancing oneself from the patient 31
9 Getting too close to the patient 33
10 The patient who refuses to talk 35

Part 2 Therapy review
11 A brief review of how drugs work 38
12 Complementary therapies 43

Part 3 The problem of pain
Some definitions of words associated with pain 52
13 Pain assessment 53
14 Treatment options for managing pain 57
15 Pain that persists or becomes out of control 63
16 Bone pain 69
17 Nerve pain 73
18 The syringe driver 78

Part 4 Common symptoms and their management
19 Abdominal swelling 88
20 Anorexia and nutrition 92
21 Bowel obstruction 99
22 Breathlessness 103
23 Cachexia 108
24 Confusion 111
25 Constipation 115
26 Cough and haemoptysis 120

27 Depression and sadness 126
28 Diarrhoea 131
29 Dysphagia 134
30 Fatigue 138
31 Fistulae 142
32 Fungating wounds 145
33 Halitosis 149
34 Hiccup 152
35 Hypercalcaemia 155
36 Itch 158
37 Jaundice 161
38 Lymphoedema 163
39 Mouth problems 167
40 Nausea and vomiting 171
41 Nightmares 177
42 Opioid-induced sedation 180
43 Skin at risk of ulceration 182
44 Sleep disorders 186
45 Spinal cord compression 188
46 Sweating 193
47 Tenesmus 196
48 Terminal restlessness 198
49 Twitching 200

Part 5 Practical issues in the care of the patient
50 Discharge planning 204
51 Where can the patient be cared for? 208
52 The family as carers 215
53 The patient is dying 220
54 Speaking to the relatives after a death 224
55 Bereavement 228

Part 6 Ethical, moral and religious issues
56 Drinking and artificial hydration (and the principles of withdrawing and withholding treatment) 232
Wilma O'Donnell
57 Refusing more treatment 237
58 Resuscitation 240
59 Spiritual and religious issues 246

Part 7 Quick practical guides
Anger and aggression: management 270
'BEFRIENDING' the patient 271
Clinical audit and clinical effectiveness 273
Communicating with deputising staff 274
Completing a death certificate 275
Dictating letters 276
Discharge prescriptions 278
End-of-life decisions 280

Genograms (family trees) 282
How good is that new drug? 283
Keeping good-quality clinical records 284
Medication chart to aid compliance 285
Mistakes and learning from them 286
Patients using the Internet as a source of information 287
Post-mortem examinations 288
Quick neurological examination 289
Reading a paper: assessing the quality of what we read 290
Recently deceased patients: a checklist 291
Reviewing a randomised controlled trial 292
Stress and relaxation 293
Supporting your colleagues 295
Teamwork and team leading 296
Working 'in TANDEM' with the patient 297
Writing a report for the coroner 298

Appendix

Useful contacts for cancer patients 300

Index **000**

Foreword

The sophistication of contemporary medical treatments for cancer leads to the expectation that the majority of individuals will continue to experience a reasonable quality of life throughout the cancer journey, and will be able to continue throughout the period of treatment with normal activities of living, and maintain key work and family responsibilities.

Despite this optimism, the majority of patients who are confronted with a diagnosis of cancer face a long, tortuous and difficult journey, marked by periods of suffering and severe debility. It is unusual for a person to travel alone on this journey. The majority of individuals are fortunate enough to have the unswerving support of immediate family, relatives and friends. This book recognises the complexity inherent in the cancer journey and places a spotlight on the human face of healthcare management, specifically on the ability to provide careful, individualised and sensitive management of symptom control that aims to make a difference to the patient's quality of life. The added value of this book is that it is written in a manner that is acceptable to professionals, patients and carers alike.

The effect of a specific treatment for a specific cancer is not consistent for all individuals, and will vary over time from one individual to another. Medical treatment is therefore affected by a range of other variables, including the person's inner strength, their ability to cope, and the social and psychological support system which they can draw upon. A significant factor in this complex journey, which is consistently voiced by patients who have experienced the long battle with cancer, is that sensitive and individualised management of the cancer journey, by experienced doctors and nurses and other key healthcare professionals, is the factor that makes a difference to the person's ability to fight, cope and ultimately survive the cancer experience.

This book demonstrates the importance of creating education resources in the field of cancer that are evidence based but also written in an inclusive style. This book is of equal value to healthcare professionals and carers who seek reliable, current, evidence-based information on the management of symptom control in a form that will help and guide them as to how best to support an individual though the cancer experience.

This book, which is intended for the non-specialist, adopts a unique approach to symptom management in palliative care, inviting the practitioner to consider the possible causes of the symptom, and then to assess the patient with these in mind. By paying attention to the pathophysiology of the symptom and respecting the individual needs of the patient, one is guided to make a logical choice of treatment by thinking about the pharmacological actions of the available drugs.

The chapter layout is the same throughout, with clear headings. This book needs to be on the desk, ready for quick reference, not sitting on a shelf in a library.

Dr Elizabeth Rogerson
Head of Education and Development,
International Virtual Nursing School (IVINURS)
Head, Distance Learning Centre
(Nursing and Palliative Care)
University of Dundee
January 2006

Preface

When we were asked about the possibility of writing this book, we were very aware that there are many textbooks on palliative care already available. To try and determine what kind of text would be useful, we undertook a survey among non-specialist doctors and nurses in several hospitals, asking what they wanted if a new book was produced.

There was a consistent request for a book that was not intended for the experienced specialist in palliative care, but for the generalist. A clear, simple and consistent layout was requested, using the same framework for each chapter so that the reader could quickly identify the section of the chapter that they wished to consult. It was requested that the text should be free from excessive references, and that it should be a book that one would use as a quick reference guide for management of common problems in palliative care, with some basic explanation of the pathophysiology and relevant pharmacology that would guide one to the most appropriate treatment.

In several of the discussions, there were requests for short guides about practical issues, and some anxiety was expressed about how to assess the value of a new treatment, how to critically read a paper, and other related issues. We have included a section at the end dealing with the topics raised. Some are not specific to the care of the cancer patient, but since they were asked for, we have included them.

Chapter headings have been kept simple, and an alphabetical layout has been used to facilitate quick and easy location of the main topics.

A four-part plan for management of patients has been adopted. The word CA℞E has been used to set out each chapter as follows.

C	**Consider** all of the patient's symptoms and all of the information available to us.
A	**Assess** the symptoms, signs and information given.
℞	**Remedy** for the problem is chosen, appropriate to the signs, symptoms and information assessed previously.
E	**Extra information** will be offered where available and appropriate.

The symbol ℞ used to appear at the top left-hand corner of all prescription pads, but has disappeared in recent years. It does not actually mean 'remedy', as we might suggest. We chose it as the word that best fits most of the applications, but is in fact derived from the Latin verb recipere, which means 'to take', and therefore in its original position it opened the prescription with the word 'take', which was followed by the details of the medications recommended by the prescriber.

The authors are aware that in choosing the title and chapter layout for this book, we have exercised a little poetic licence with regard to the use and interpretation of the ℞ symbol where our recommendations follow, from which we invite you to take anything that is useful.

The principles of clinical governance will be applied throughout, encouraging best clinical practice, and where possible an evidence-based approach will be adopted, recognising the difficulties associated with conducting good-quality randomised controlled trials in patients suffering from cancer.

It must be remembered that it is difficult to obtain good evidence for some of the treatments suggested, and some reports of their use are, of necessity, based on the experiences of others in respected centres. In palliative care, some drugs are used outside of their licence. No evidence will be available for this situation, but the suggestions included are tried and tested and have been proved to be effective, even though the pharmacology remains unclear.

We have tried to use standard and readily available journals for the suggested further reading. Some topics are extensively covered in the journals, others less so. This is reflected in the individual chapters. Referencing in the text has been kept to a minimum by listing the resource texts we used at the beginning of the book (*see* page xiii).

Wesley C Finegan
Angela McGurk
January 2007

About the authors

Wesley C Finegan MB BCh, BAO, MRCGP, MICGP, D Pall Med
Wesley studied medicine at Queen's University in Belfast, qualifying in 1978. He spent 10 years in general practice, during which time he became increasingly involved in palliative care, and this resulted in him changing jobs and being appointed as consultant in palliative medicine in 1991.

In 1994, Wesley developed cancer and had to retire from clinical practice, but he continues to work in medical education and teaching on palliative care programmes.

He has written two earlier books, *Trust Me; I'm a ~~Doctor~~ Cancer Patient* (2004) and *Being a Cancer Patient's Carer: a guide* (2005), both published by Radcliffe Publishing. The latter title won the Society of Authors and Royal Society of Medicine prize for first-edition medical books for the general reader, and was highly commended in the British Medical Association medical book competition in the popular medicine section.

In July 2006, Wesley was given the award of Graduate of the Year by Queen's University Belfast in recognition of his second book, written while caring for his wife Alice, who died of cancer in August 2005.

Angela McGurk RGN, Dip Ed
Angela trained as a nurse at Stobhill Hospital, Glasgow, qualifying in 1982. She went on to complete a Diploma in Higher Education, in caring for the older person, at the University of York.

She has spent her career working in acute medicine and older people's services. Throughout her career she has cared for people with palliative care needs.

Angela now works for Southern Cross Healthcare as a care home manager in Glenrothes.

Wilma O'Donnell BSc, PG Dip in Palliative Nursing Care, SPQ, ENP, SP, RGN
Wilma, who trained at Forth Valley College of Nursing and qualified in 1982, is a palliative care specialist nurse who works as part of a hospital palliative care team within the acute sector.

The main component of her workload is symptom management, which includes support for patients, families and staff throughout the cancer journey.

Jan Pederson RGN, DN
Jan trained at Redhill General Hospital, qualifying in 1970. She worked as a ward sister in gynaecology, care of the elderly and also intensive therapy and coronary care before training to become a district nurse in 1986. She worked in the out-of-hours community palliative care service for about six years, and continued her interest in palliative care later as a district nurse with extensive input into a local palliative care home team led by local GPs.

Jan moved into practice nursing in 1988, gained Specialist Practitioner status in 1998 and qualified as a District Nurse Prescriber two years later. She has recently extended her skills and is now a fully Independent Nurse Prescriber. Her special interests include women's health, diabetes, travel health and asthma.

Acknowledgements

This book was requested to meet the needs of non-specialist doctors and nurses who have to deal with and manage patients with cancer-related symptoms.

We wish to thank those who asked for the book to be written, and the various doctors and nurses who have read individual chapters and provided feedback and guidance to help us to provide the kind of information they want, in a suitable format.

We also thank the many patients who have taught us over the years, and whose experiences have helped us to increase our knowledge and experience in managing their problems.

Thanks are due to Wilma O'Donnell and Jan Pederson for their written contributions, and to Sandra Campbell and Liz MacMillan for guidance, advice and suggestions.

We wish to express our gratitude to John, Kerryann and Megan for their patience.

Finally, we thank the staff of Radcliffe Publishing for their guidance, advice and support throughout the various stages in the production of this text.

Resource texts

In an attempt to make the text as easy to read as possible, we have tried to keep references to a minimum and as specific as possible. The books listed below were consulted frequently and used as resource material for various chapters.

- BMA and Royal Pharmaceutical Society of Great Britain. *British National Formulary*. London: BMA and Royal Pharmaceutical Society of Great Britain; 2006.
- Charlton R, editor. *Primary Palliative Care*. Oxford: Radcliffe Medical Press; 2002.
- Doyle D, Hanks GW, Cherny NI *et al. The Oxford Textbook of Palliative Medicine*. Oxford: Oxford University Press; 2004.
- McCaffery M, Pasero C. *Pain: clinical manual*. St Louis, MO: Mosby; 1999.
- Morrison RS, Meier DE. *Geriatric Palliative Care*. Oxford: Oxford University Press; 2003.
- Regnard C, Hockley J. *A Guide to Symptom Relief in Palliative Care*. Oxford: Radcliffe Publishing; 2004.
- Summerhayes M, Daniels S. *Practical Chemotherapy*. Oxford: Radcliffe Medical Press; 2003.
- Thomas K. *Caring for the Dying at Home*. Oxford: Radcliffe Medical Press; 2003.
- Twycross R, Wilcock A, Charlesworth S *et al. Palliative Care Formulary 2*. Oxford: Radcliffe Medical Press; 2002.
- Watson M, Lucas C, Hoy A *et al. Oxford Handbook of Palliative Care*. Oxford: Oxford University Press; 2005.

What standards of treatment and care can the patient reasonably expect?

In the spring of 2004, the National Institute for Clinical Excellence (NICE) published a document called *Guidance on Cancer Services: improving supportive and palliative care in adults with cancer.*[1]

In summary, the document reminds us that patients can reasonably expect:

1 to be involved in decision making
2 staff to communicate clearly with them
3 the members of the caring team to communicate clearly with each other
4 to be given the name of a staff member whom they can contact for help and advice
5 to be given as much information as they want
6 to have their social and practical needs addressed in addition to their medical and physical problems
7 to have their emotional and spiritual needs recognised and addressed
8 to be offered appropriate help and rehabilitation to help them to live with the effects of cancer
9 to have their families and other carers recognised as important, and for them to be offered appropriate emotional and practical support, especially at times of diagnosis and bereavement
10 to be offered a quick response at times of greatest need when their disease is progressing rapidly
11 to have their preference about their place of death respected, and recognition given to their wishes about continuation of treatment
12 to be involved in making cancer services better by having their voice heard in patient forums.

These are recommendations, not rights, but they do set reasonable standards of care that we can all try to achieve.

Reference

1 National Institute for Clinical Excellence. *Guidance on Cancer Services: improving supportive and palliative care in adults with cancer.* London: National Institute for Clinical Excellence; 2004.
Two versions of these recommendations on cancer care in England and Wales are available – a shorter version for the public and a full version for healthcare professionals. Both are available to download from the NICE website (www.nice.org.uk), or by telephoning 0870 155 5455, quoting N0474 for the full version or N0476 for the shorter guide.

Further reading

- Cates C. Finding the evidence – where to look for answers. *Prescriber.* 2002; **13:** 47–50.
- Donald J. GMS indicators set baseline for care of patients with cancer. *Guidelines Pract.* 2004; **7:** 32–8.
- Drew A, Fawcett TN. Responding to the information needs of patients with cancer. *Prof Nurse.* 2002; **17**: 443–6.
- Greenhalgh T. *How to Read a Paper: the basics of evidence-based medicine.* London: BMJ Publishing Group; 1997.
- Harris D, Richard B, Khanna P. Palliative care for the elderly: a need unmet. *Geriatr Med.* 2006; **36:** 29–33.
- Hermet R, Burucoa B, Sentilhes-Monkham A. The need for evidence-based proof in palliative care. *Eur J Palliat Care.* 2002; **9:** 104–7.
- Higginson IJ. Evidence-based palliative care? *Eur J Palliat Care.* 1999; **6:** 188–93.
- Joyce L. Translating knowledge into good practice. *Prof Nurse.* 2000; **16:** 960–63.
- Payne S. Information needs of patients and families. *Eur J Palliat Care.* 2002; **9:** 112–14.
- Thomas K. Palliative care. *Geriatr Med.* 2006; **36:** 9–13. (This paper includes a discussion of the Gold Standards Framework and the NHS End-of-Life Care Programme.)
- Thomas K, Free A. The Gold Standards Framework is pivotal to palliative care. *Guidelines Pract.* 2006; **9:** 29–40.

Part 1

Communicating with the patient

Chapter 1

Basic issues in communication

All around my bed is a great big curtain;
There's someone there behind it, but I don't know who.
It sounds to me like doctors, but I can't be certain,
And specialists and nurses, too.
They're talking very quietly and muttering together
About the need for surgery, or therapy, or what.
It all sounds pretty dodgy, and I don't know whether
I'm the subject of their little plot.

Christopher Matthew[1]

Introduction

Much has been written on the subject of communication with cancer patients, and many training courses are available, which serves to highlight the importance of this topic.

There are a number of issues that can arise when we are speaking to patients. These include the following possible problems:

- anger
- collusion
- confidentiality issues
- denial
- distancing oneself from the patient
- getting too close to the patient
- refusal to talk.

C Consider

What are the perceived problems with our communication skills when dealing with cancer patients?

Patients sometimes say that:

- they were told too little
- they were told too much
- they were told too quickly
- they were not able to understand what was said
- they did not believe what they were told.

A Assess

- What does the patient already *know* about their illness and prognosis?
- Who gave the patient this information?
- How accurate is this information?

Be aware of the risk that patients may sometimes quote verbatim what was said to them. Does this mean that they understood the message and its implications? We can teach parrots to recite sentences accurately, but they don't necessarily understand the meaning!

℞ Remedy

It is important to establish 'common ground' before entering into further discussion, especially when one has bad news to impart.

- Find out, preferably in their own words, exactly what the patient knows about their diagnosis, their expectations of the treatment available and their prognosis.
- How much do they want to know now and how quickly do they wish to be told?

There are some basic 'rules' that can be quickly summarised as follows.

Ambiguity must be avoided at all costs. Use language that your patient understands.

Check the patient's understanding by asking them to summarise the conversation in their own words. Repetition of phrases does not prove understanding of the message.

In this respect, let us share a true story. WF was attending an outpatient clinic as a patient when this happened.

An elderly Scottish woman emerged from the consultant's room beaming with happiness. She approached WF and said 'What a lovely doctor and what good news he gave me. He is going to give me the "cream o'therapy". Poor you, you'll only be getting the milk!'

Before WF had an opportunity to explain that she might have misunderstood the term 'chemotherapy', the patient had scuttled out of the waiting room.

As a patient, what was WF's responsibility?

Cue-based questions like 'What was that like for you?' can invite open honest sharing.

Listening can be active or passive.

- 'Active' listening involves eye contact and appropriate body language to encourage the patient to talk.
- 'Passive' listening offers less of your attention, and patients may tend to say less.

Note taking is essential, but patients may think that you are paying less attention to them. Agree with the patient that you may take notes, why you are taking them and who else may see them (assure them of the confidentiality of the notes that are written), and let them see that you are still giving them your full attention.

Observe the patient. Do their verbal and non-verbal messages say the same things?

Questions should be 'open' to encourage the patient to offer the information in their own words. 'Closed' questions have only one possible answer (e.g. 'What is your date of birth?'). These do not encourage the patient to 'open up' and talk freely. Leading questions should be avoided, as they often result in biased answers intended to please the person who is asking.

Summarise the consultation at the end, making sure that the patient has taken in what you were saying.

Time is always the enemy! No matter how much time you have, the patient may think you are too busy to talk. Reassure them if you have time to have a full discussion. If not, agree a mutually acceptable time for a return visit to discuss the issues in depth.

Another anecdote. WF was attending for radiotherapy. An elderly woman emerged from the treatment room and saw him sitting outside.

'Do I look all right?' she asked in a conspiratorial whisper.

WF, recognising that he is a mere man, assured the lady that she looked fine.

'I don't glow, do I?'

'No, why should you?'

'All I know about radium is that my husband used a special paint to paint the instrument dials on war planes. I think it contained radium and the paint glowed green in the dark.'

'I don't glow in the dark, so you won't either.'

'That's good. I just wondered. He did great work. He used to suck his paint-brush to get a nice fine point to do fine work. Poor love died of cancer of the tongue. I don't know how, for he never smoked.'

On this occasion, because WF knew both the radiographers treating him, he recounted this story. The staff admitted that, due to pressure of time, the woman had not received an explanation of the treatment schedule, nor had she had the opportunity to discuss any fears or anxieties.

Before we criticise, however, remember that we all live in the real world. Don't we all face the same enemy – time, or lack of it?

Use the concept of working in TANDEM with the patient to help them to think about the questions they might wish to ask now or at a later time (*see* page 297). This allows them some control over how much they are told and how quickly they have to come to terms with the information.

E Extra information

It is a well-documented fact that on hearing the word 'cancer', the shock can be such that the rest of the conversation is lost and the patient may subsequently deny having been given significant pieces of information.[2] Interviews have been taped so that the patient and their family can listen to them afterwards. Patients may complain that they were actually told too much, but at least this technique allows them to listen at their own pace, and to listen more than once, and it also avoids any misunderstanding or inaccurate reporting by the patient and their relatives about what was actually said.[3]

It is of interest that the use of taped interviews in a general practice setting increased patient recall, improved satisfaction with the treatment offered and helped patients to share the information with others involved in their care. However, it did not have any effect on adherence to the advice given or on anxiety associated with the presenting problem.[4]

References

1 Matthew C. 'Touch and go.' In: *Now We Are Sixty (And A Bit)*. London: John Murray; 2003.
2 Fallowfield LJ, Baum M, Maguire GP. Effects of breast conservation on psychological morbidity associated with diagnosis and treatment of early breast cancer. *BMJ*. 1986; **293:** 1331–4.
3 Hogbin BJ, Fallowfield LJ. Getting it taped: the 'bad news' consultation in a general surgical department. *Br J Hosp Med*. 1988; **41:** 330–33.
4 Liddell C *et al.* Giving patients an audiotape of their GP consultation: a randomised controlled trial. *Br J Gen Pract*. 2004; **54:** 667–72.

Further reading

- Brewin T, Sparshott M. *Relating to the Relatives*. Oxford: Radcliffe Medical Press; 1996.
- Campbell S. A project to promote better communication with patients. *Nurs Times*. 2006; **102:** 28–30.
- Hobma S *et al.* Effective improvement of doctor–patient communication: a randomised controlled trial. *Br J Gen Pract*. 2006; **56:** 580–86.
- Kirk P, Kirk I, Kristjanson LJ. What do patients receiving palliative care for cancer and their families want to be told? A Canadian and Australian qualitative study. *BMJ*. 2004; **328:** 1343–7.
- Lugton J. *Communicating with Dying People and Their Relatives*. Oxford: Radcliffe Medical Press; 2002.
- Sheldon F, Oliviere D. Family information and communication – what works? *Eur J Palliat Care*. 2005; **12:** 254–6.
- Surbone A, Zwitter M. Communication with the cancer patient: information and truth. *Ann N Y Acad Sci*. 1997; **809**. (This is a 500 page+ volume devoted to this subject, dealing with virtually every culture worldwide.)

Chapter 2

Listening effectively: 'ALWAYS REACT'

Jan Pederson

> One of the best pieces of advice ever given to doctors, nurses or other health workers is that each time they see a patient, they ask themselves two questions.
> 1 What can I do for this patient?
> 2 What can I learn from this patient?
> There is always something to do and there is always something to learn.
>
> Anon.[1]

Introduction

There is so much more to listening than just the verbal messages that the patient gives us. Everyone constantly sends out non-verbal signals, and effective assessment involves picking up the cues and also being aware of our own 'non-verbal leakages' of emotions and feelings.

Some years ago, when working as a district nurse with one of the authors (WF), I became fascinated by the vast numbers of simple but easily overlooked non-verbal signals that are being transmitted but frequently missed.

We agreed that it is only when you 'always listen with all your senses' that these have any hope of being picked up, whether it is appropriate to deal with them or not at the time. We agreed to try to do this – 'always,' We were amazed both by the things we had missed and by the non-verbal messages that we ourselves might be transmitting.

This is a huge subject, and I can only scratch the surface layer, but here are some thoughts for you to build on. There are so many areas of overlap that some repetition or omission is almost unavoidable.

I write as an English girl born and bred, but we need to be aware of the ethnic, religious and cultural differences, and to respect individual and personal feelings and beliefs. I noted the following comment:

> Modern medicine is certainly not a folklore festival, and nice words about the rich diversity of cultures may sound idealistic. No matter how unusual some of the beliefs, rituals and sociological patterns may be to an outsider, the physician cannot ignore the patient's cultural background and his or her support network.[2]

C Consider

It is the right of our patients to have privacy, and sometimes they deliberately withhold information for one reason or another. Much more often, however, they might be wishing to say something, but fear, embarrassment or simple inability to recognise what needs to be said means that some important message remains unmentioned and is therefore not assessed, and therefore a need remains unaddressed.

If we can improve our skills in picking up these non-verbal cues, we can invite discussion on the subject and, if this is refused, we know that the patient is not ready to explore that area, but at least it was not missed, leaving the patient suffering in silence.

A Assess

We all have the same five basic senses – sight, hearing, smell, taste and touch. We must use these as we enter each consultation, in whatever setting, as each sense gives us important clues and pointers to the whole patient, their environment and their needs.

Sight

This is our first assessment on arrival, and it can start outside the house in a community setting. What do the garden and the general exterior tell us? Is there a handrail for disability, an unkempt garden or signs of recent or long-term inability to cope?

On entry, is there unopened mail on the floor, a newspaper not taken in, and other signs that things are being left until later because of weakness, inability or simple lack of interest and motivation?

What do we see next? These lists cannot possibly be exhaustive!

The patient

- Appearance – clean, tidy, washed, unkempt, nutritional state, weight change, etc.
- Demeanour – depressed, disinterested, dismal, distant, dour, down, etc.
- Eyes – bright and shiny, happy, sad, dull and sagging from pain or lack of sleep. Does the patient make eye contact at all? We can learn a phenomenal amount from a patient's eyes, and they have little control over this very honest form of non-verbal communication. Think about their visual acuity as well. Do they seem to be able to get about without risk and should they be driving?
- Physical signs – everything from finger clubbing to a fungating wound comes to mind. Look for and take note of the signs of disease – the fine tremor that is so easily missed, the coarse skin and dry hair of hypothyroidism, the exophthalmos of thyrotoxicosis, or even just the signs of nicotine staining that do not match the patient's verbal admission of how much they smoke.
- Sexuality and body image. Patients will probably not raise this topic, but that is no reason not to be aware of what you see and the effect that it is having on the patient's personal and interpersonal relationships. Does the patient feel rejected, repulsive or revolting due to a fungating wound or some other onslaught on body image?

The environment

There is so much here, but a few starters are listed below.

- Cleaning. Is the house tidy, untidy or dirty?
- Clothing. Is there evidence of not keeping up to date with personal or domestic laundry?
- Companion animals. Are they cared for, or a risk to the patient?
- Cooking. Is the patient at nutritional risk? What about meal provision? Look for unfinished meals, half-drunk cups of tea, or perhaps no evidence of drinking adequate fluids at all. Perhaps the patient is drinking, but not tea and coffee! Look for signs of alcohol use.
- Coping. Is there evidence that the patient needs to be cared for in another way or in another place?
- Clutter. Is there junk lying around? This may be normal, but one can pick up some clues to this. Are there unopened newspaper or letters? Do these indicate an inability to read due to a visual problem, or just a lack of interest, energy or motivation?

These can be missed, and some patients carefully disguise the signs. WF and I visited an elderly, very proud woman whose home was immaculate and whose bedroom gave no indication that she and her husband actually used separate rooms, which explained how she hid a fungating breast tumour for months until she became so distressed by the pain and odour that she was forced to seek attention.

Hearing

What do we hear as we approach the patient? Are there sounds or silence? If there are sounds, what are they? Are they appropriate, explained and expected, or do they ring alarm bells in our minds? If there is silence, does this indicate that the patient is unaware of our approach, just naturally quiet or too fed up to speak?

A few brainstormed thoughts are listed below, to which you can add your own.

- Accents. Simple, but easily overlooked, and either party may misunderstand the other as a result of a simple change in pronunciation.
- Companion animals. Are they constantly barking and creating a communication barrier? Don't forget hearing dogs for hearing-impaired people.
- Deafness. This is often carefully disguised due to embarrassment.
- Distractions. Our modern society is invaded by background noise, so deal with a radio, television, mobile phones or loud music permeating from the teenager's bedroom if necessary. Avoid taking phone calls during consultations.
- Family and friends can be there to listen and reinforce the message later, or may add to the risk of loss of confidentiality. Ask the patient how they feel about their presence.
- Language. Language and cultural differences in how we communicate verbally and non-verbally are always relevant.
- Laughter. This is the very best medicine. Yes, it is allowed, with the patient's permission, and it can take the consultation on to a new and more efficient level.

- Lip reading. How many of our patients partially lip read, not because they are deaf as such, but because they have a significant enough loss, possibly due to something simple like ear wax? They can only lip read if they can see your lips!
- Music. During long or painful procedures, or while having chemotherapy, patients may find music relaxing, and it might aid and facilitate conversation. Invite the patient to bring their own choice of tape or CD. Your choice of relaxing Mozart and their choice of Phil Collins may be quite different, but they will appreciate the 'control' offered by this simple choice. Be aware of the fact that some people like their music loud. Did we not all study with the stereo at full volume? It is not always seen as a problem by the person who likes this level of input. You might like music while you work, but be aware of the distraction it may be to the patient.
- Selective hearing. We all know patients do this, but which bit was selected?
- Silence. Silence speaks volumes. It takes time to allow bad news to sink in. If the silence is becoming a barrier and the patient is refusing to talk, this needs to be dealt with, but a short reflective silence is allowed and is normal and natural.
- Speech. Who is doing all the talking? Are you saying too much at one time? What is the content of what is being said by the patient?
- Sweet smiles and nods. We have all been there with the patient who non-verbally seemed to agree with every word and left looking composed and content, but was in fact confused, completely unaware of what was said and heard almost nothing.
- Trivialities. Be alert for the phrase 'I didn't want to bother you with this'. It is usually bothering the patient a lot more than they wish to admit. They may only be seeking reassurance, but it requires a proper investigation so that you don't miss something, even though they thought it too minor to bother you about!

Smell

Smells fall into two simple categories, pleasant and unpleasant. We all have individual preferences, and we find that aromas arouse memories and are associated with a variety of emotions and experiences.

Unpleasant smells

Some of the unpleasant smells that we associate with care of cancer patients include the following.

- Air 'fresheners'. These usually serve only to remind us that one smell is being partly replaced with another. Our immediate thought is to wonder what is being masked and if there is not a better way to deal with it in the first place.
- Animal aromas. Is there evidence of companion animals whose care is less than optimal, due to failing health and increasing inability to attend to the animal's needs?
- Cooking smells. These can be very intolerable to a nauseous patient.

- Fungating wounds such as a breast carcinoma. I well recall my first experience of this when I was a first-year student nurse. A patient in her forties was admitted with a fungating breast carcinoma which she had kept from her husband for months by sleeping in the spare room, using the excuse that she was worried her snoring would keep him awake! She was petrified of going to the doctor. She only lived for a few more days. I shall never forget that smell. Nor will I ever forget her. She taught me so much, although I didn't realise it at the time.
- Incontinence. This is usually fairly obvious, and requires sensitive but early attention.
- Musty and unkept house. Again, this is fairly easy to spot and should prompt discussion and appropriate action to help the patient to cope, with whatever input is needed.
- Sweat. The sweating may well be due to pain, intense fear, anger, inability to be self-caring or, sadly, laziness. Whatever the cause, it can be a barrier to being tactile and one must work hard to disguise feelings of revulsion if someone or something smells unpleasant.
- Urine. This may be due to incontinence, prostate trouble or inconvenient toilet facilities, among other causes.

Pleasant smells

- Bed linen. What patient does not enjoy a fresh crisp pleasantly scented new sheet on the bed?
- Cooking. An appetising cooking smell, such as bread baking, is so pleasant and gives the impression of being in control, in charge and making healthy food.
- Fresh flowers. These are always welcome unless one is allergic to pollen! Or are they? One relative commented that the scent of the flowers was a reminder of her father's illness. She hated it being there every time his condition deteriorated, because it happened repeatedly and made it more real and harder for her to accept.

And how often do we smell something and relive a childhood memory? Is it always a positive association?

Taste

Here I am using a little poetic licence and borrowing my husband John's thought and using the word 'flavour' as well. We expose our patients to so many unwanted flavours, and many of the treatments that we offer result in a bad taste in their mouths. A few random thoughts are listed below.

- Altered taste. During illness, or as a result of chemotherapy or radiotherapy, the patient may be experiencing an alteration in how foods taste. One patient described having a fishy taste in his mouth for 18 weeks while he was on chemotherapy for a lymphoma. Many patients experience a metallic taste while on medication.
- Compliance (concordance). Is it any wonder that patients may not fully comply with taking a foul-tasting medicine? Lactulose is so sweet, morphine is so bitter, and senna – well, disgusting is the only word!

- Dry mouth. Many drugs cause a dry mouth, as does head and neck radiotherapy. Without saliva, taste is seriously altered or absent.
- Flavours. We all have our preferences, our likes and dislikes, but who can blame one patient who now never eats fish after 18 weeks of tasting nothing else? There is a supermarket he told me about where the fish counter is by the entrance. He shops in a more expensive and less convenient store because the smell of fish brings back memories which are so strongly associated with the treatment that he cannot even enter the premises.
- Olfactory hallucinations. High doses of dexamethasone cause olfactory hallucinations in some patients. One patient described smelling something like an aromatic air freshener all the time, saying to me that 'the smell of aromatic oils, mixed with a good peppered steak, is beyond imagination'.

The simplest tastes can be 'nectar'. That fresh glass of cold water after an operation or having one's first baby! And what would life be without chocolate?

Touch

Desmond Morris, in his book *Intimate Behaviour*, states that 'We often talk about the way we talk, and we frequently try to see the way we see, but for some reason we have rarely touched on the way we touch'.[3]

I have always been told I'm a very tactile person, whatever that means. I would naturally offer my hand, touch and feel comfortable to do so, but what does the patient perceive in this? Again a series of thoughts come to mind, but you will be able to add many others.

- Barriers caused by gloves. When I trained, we wore gloves so little compared with today, when we seem to be wearing them almost constantly. When we touched someone, it was skin-to-skin contact complete with all the tactile sensations we pick up in our sensitive nerve endings in our finger tips. The barrier of vinyl deprives us of a sense of the temperature or texture of skin, moistness and clamminess, and even some of the bonding that touch should achieve.
- The colour of the skin is so revealing. Cyanosis, pigmentation or lack of pigmentation, nicotine stains, and so on, all come to mind. One patient once appeared with brown stains on his hands and, knowing that he was a non-smoker, these aroused my interest. He was having chemotherapy for cancer, and had developed bleomycin staining which was so similar in colour to tobacco staining that I wondered what his friends might have thought if they had not known better. It could have been so easy to assume, to get it wrong and even to cause offence.
- Disease. The coolness, clamminess, sweatiness or other signs, like a fine tremor, or loss of grip or coordination, are all there to be picked up when we touch by simply shaking hands.
- Environmental factors. Compare the temperature of the skin with the ambient temperature. Is there a difference? Is the skin too hot, or too cold?
- Examinations using gloves. These are essential, but they represent a barrier, as already mentioned.
- Hand holding. Does the patient indicate that they see it as a sign of weakness if they cry or accept a gentle gesture? As someone said recently, saying

verbally that one is 'fine' can be an acronym for 'Feeling In Need of Encouragement', but they simply cannot admit this openly. This is not only true of men, as might easily be assumed. We must also be sensitive to the way in which gestures are interpreted by patients and staff of the opposite sex. In addition, we should be aware of cultural differences in the use of gestures.

- Hands-on approach. I am always very conscious of making sure that my hands are as smooth as possible. I've always said that I much prefer to be 'hands on'. However, that isn't much good if your skin is dry and rough. Similarly, if a patient's skin is rough, what does this tell us? Do they have eczema or psoriasis? Do they have a manual job?
- Handshake. The handshake of greeting tells so much. Grip, temperature and texture of skin can all be instantly assessed. Is the hand offered confidently and enthusiastically, with accurate coordination? Or is there a fumbling half-hearted response to your greeting? Does the patient make eye contact? What does that non-verbal sign tell you? Do the signs match?
- Occupational factors. Hands tell us a lot about a person's job. Does the skin texture match your understanding of how their hands should feel?
- Reactions to touch. When you touch someone who is not so tactile, what if you misread the signals and they pull away? Are they telling you (or themselves) that they can cope without your interventions? Perhaps they are afraid of showing emotion.
- Skin disorders. The skin provides such an accurate reflection of inner health, and so many illnesses have dermatological signs. Observe and associate them.
- Skin temperature is important. Vascular disorders, fever and hypothermia are just a few of the signs we are offered so readily here. My mother tells me off every time I visit because of my cold hands. They are actually quite nice on your forehead if you've got a fever!
- Stroking a companion animal is well documented as a means of controlling blood pressure and helping us to relax. Can bonding with the companion animal help us to bond with the patient as well?
- Tactile versus 'no touch' personalities. So much comfort is derived from being held or putting your arms around someone. But does the patient feel safe in this embrace? We need to be aware of how our patients feel.

> To touch is not a technique: not touching is a technique.
>
> J Older[4]

℞ Remedy

I've just been baking bread. The wonderful smell is permeating the entire house. I hope it will taste good. I've just heard the timer ring to remind me it's ready. I must be careful not to burn my fingers when I take it from the oven to touch/feel the texture. It looks good enough to eat!

John has walked into the kitchen and is obviously ready to try my loaf. It occurred to me that I was watching him react to the sight and smell of my new loaf. I said so, and he replied 'I Respond Effectively As my Conscience Tells'. Bless him, he has just given me a new acronym.

As I watched him, I recognised that we REACT with all our senses as well. I was aware of his delight when he saw the loaf. He showed pleasure in the smell of the freshly baked bread. He is picking bits off to sample and obviously enjoying the texture and flavour, making sounds of appreciation.

How do we react? We 'ALWAYS REACT' to every situation in some way. What do we give away? Do we wrinkle our noses, gulp, gasp, hold our breath, retch, smile, look excited, or what?

We may be saying one thing verbally but conveying or meaning something completely different with our body language – our accent, tone, delays in replying, hesitation in choosing the right word. The list is endless.

We taste the situation, getting the flavour of things, or balancing out information from our own senses to make a call (on the flavour of things) on how best to help. We may offer:

- proactive help – leading down a particular path
- reactive help – guiding down a particular path.

We judge what we should offer. For example, we look at the strong person, possibly with a need to guide them. However, if we try to lead, they are more likely to go against what we are saying. We look at the weak person and see our need to lead. However, if we try to guide rather than lead, a weak person may be more likely to fall.

We empathise, putting ourselves in someone else's position, knowing how they feel. This gives us a flavour of their demeanour and how they are feeling. The more we can empathise, the better we can help with and/or advise about a person's needs.

Does our body language show interest, enthusiasm, apathy, or what?

Do our faces show something that we try to hide in our spoken replies?

No matter how we try, we are making a judgement call or assessment by always listening with all our senses, and the way in which we react is being monitored by our patients, who will spend hours analysing every verbal reply and our non-verbal leakage of information and emotion.

As well as listening *with* all of our senses, we also must listen *to* all of our senses and be aware of how we are coming across to our patients.

Our senses are so powerful. We could not communicate or express ourselves without them. Memories relate to past experiences that stimulated all our senses. What happens, then, if they are taken away?

E Extra information

The Bible states that 'what has been will be again, what has been done will be done again; there is nothing new under the sun' (Ecclesiastes, Chapter 1, verse 9).

While researching this chapter, I found a picture, dating from around 1485, showing physicians examining the urine of a pregnant woman. The text accompanying the picture reminds us that the medieval medics:

- listened to the patient's breathing
- looked at the skin colour
- smelt for gangrene

- tasted the urine
- touched the wrist to feel the pulse.

In other words, over 500 years ago, they 'always listened with all their senses.' There is indeed 'nothing new under the sun'.

References

1 Found on the Internet in a series of medical quotations. Original source not identified.
2 Surbone A, Zwitter M. Communicating with the cancer patient. *Ann N Y Acad Sci.* 1997; **809:** 3.
3 Morris D. *Intimate Behaviour*. London: Book Club Associates; 1971.
4 Older J. *Touching is Healing*. New York: Stein & Day Publishers; 1982.

Further reading

- Autton N. *Touch: an exploration*. London: Darton, Longman and Todd; 1989.
- Helman CG. Doctor–patient interactions. In: *Culture, Health and Illness*. Oxford: Butterworth Heinemann; 2000.

Chapter 3

Breaking bad news

> In the presence of the patient, Latin is the language.
>
> Medieval maxim

Introduction

Giving a patient the news of a terminal illness, a poor prognosis, or telling them that they have cancer is never easy. It does not get any easier with time and experience. There may be individual feelings of inadequacy, anxiety about how the news will be received, and fear of doing it wrong. Some teams have policies about what is said, when and how, all of which can make a difficult job even harder.

C Consider

- What does the patient already know?
- Where are they in their illness?

Patients are often suspicious, but have not had their fears formally confirmed. They will be understandably anxious. Anxiety is not conducive to absorbing what is being said. As well as 'where they are' and how much they know, you need to consider the following:

- how much does the patient want to know? Will they be confident to ask when they wish to know more?
- think about cultural traditions with regard to breaking bad news. In Japan, for example, it is traditional to tell the relatives but to 'protect' the patient. Does the patient want to be told?
- is there any impairment to the patient hearing the news? This could be due to a sensory loss, a language difficulty or poor memory.
- how much time can you offer now? Can you deal with all of the issues adequately at this consultation?
- is there a specialist nurse who can be present who can be available for the patient to speak to later, to confirm what was said and answer any questions that arise? Does the patient wish this nurse or another person to be present now?

A Assess

How much can the patient take in now? Acknowledge their anxiety about being given bad news that they possibly didn't expect.

Assess how far they can go in this interview and how soon you need to meet to take this interview forward.

℞ Remedy

Bad news is always bad news, however skilled one is in imparting it. Some basic 'rules' always apply.

- Confidentiality is vital. Find a private place for the discussion – a curtain round the bed is not adequate.
- Do not rush the interview. Patients are very aware of the constraints on staff time, and often will not ask questions that really need to be answered now.
- Prepare the patient. Give a warning that there is bad news to follow, and let that sink in before proceeding.
- Time is needed for adjusting to the news. Give the patient facts at a pace appropriate to their ability to take them in and absorb the news.

Patients often give the impression that they are coping with the news they have been given. This may be an attempt to appear calm and coping, so always remember the following points.

- Acknowledge their difficulty in accepting the truth of what is being said and deal with their disbelief, disappointment and shock at what they have been told.
- Assess the patient's verbal and non-verbal responses. Are they compatible?
- Expect questions and answer them honestly. If you don't know all the answers, say so. Explain if there may be answers later when more facts are known, with more test results, etc. Give some idea of when you might have more information and answers. Remember that time drags very slowly if you are an anxious patient awaiting results!

There are a couple of commonly made mistakes that are easily avoided.

- Avoid giving bad news and then immediately starting to talk in detail about 'treatment', as this just causes confusion. The term 'treatment' implies hope of a cure. This may not be a realistic expectation, and you do not want to generate false hope. Allow time for one message to sink in before moving on.
- Don't be tempted to automatically give advice as soon as you are asked a question. Sometimes we need time to find out the full answer. If so, explain this and agree a time to meet and discuss the matter further. Remember, time passes very slowly for patients who want results or information!

E Extra information

A number of methods have been suggested for breaking bad news. One of these is the 'SPIKES' model suggested by Beale *et al.*[1] This model uses a six-step approach, as summarised below.

Step 1 S Setting up the interview

- Arrange adequate privacy.
- Allow the patient to invite and involve significant others.
- Sit down, as this implies that you have time to talk.
- Connect with the patient – make eye contact and touch them if appropriate.
- Manage your time and try to avoid interruptions.

Step 2 P Patient's perception

- Use open-ended questions to assess what the patient already knows and understands about their illness, treatment and prognosis. Adopt an 'ask before you tell' approach.
- Use this information to correct any misconceptions, and as a basis for tailoring your message to the patient.

Step 3 I Invite the patient to discuss their situation with you

- Most patients will welcome any opportunity to learn about their illness and ask questions, but some will not want to talk. Don't force them before they are ready.
- Being asked for information may make the 'bad news' interview a little easier, but be aware of those patients who are coping by denial and don't want to hear anything that challenges this defence mechanism.
- If they do not want to be told about the illness as such, at least invite them to ask any questions they might have.

Step 4 K Knowledge and information given to the patient

- The first piece of knowledge the patient needs is a warning that there is bad news to come.
- Give the patient information at a pace and in amounts appropriate to their ability to understand and take in what is being said. Go at the pace set by the patient, and build on their existing knowledge and understanding as already assessed.
- Use simple terms like 'disease has spread' rather than 'metastasised', and 'tissue sample' rather than 'biopsy'. Words like 'ulcer' can also be misunderstood and may be thought to imply a non-malignant process.
- Be honest in a sensitive way, but not blunt. Bluntness can result in anger, perceived lack of concern and a sense of isolation.
- Check regularly that the message is being understood and retained, as it is easy to overload the patient with facts.
- Even when the prognosis is bad, there is always something that can be done. Cure may not be possible, but care is always possible. Never say that there is 'nothing more that can be done', as patients then lose hope. Explain that there is no cure possible, but that you (or the palliative care team) will be there for the patient and their family through the illness and for the relatives and others through the period of bereavement. Choose your time and words carefully. These are difficult concepts to take on board.

Step 5 E Emotional assessment

The common reactions to unexpected bad news are disbelief, anger and denial, possibly associated with crying or silence. Sometimes patients are relieved to have an explanation for the symptoms they have reported, but there may be anger over a perceived delay in the diagnosis, associated with the thought that an earlier diagnosis might have offered hope of a better outcome. These thoughts should be explored honestly and fully, because they will persist and may lead to a lack of trust in the team if incorrect perceptions are not corrected. If there has been late presentation or a delay in diagnosis, the reasons for this should be explored and explained honestly.

Whatever the reaction, there are some basic steps to follow.

- Observe and record the patient's emotional reaction, including anger, denial, despair, tears, etc.
- Ask what they think and feel about the news they have just been given, and record their response. Silence may be the only response you get!
- Is the response appropriate? Is the reason obvious and identifiable? Is anger justified? Against whom is it directed?
- Acknowledge the emotional response and the diagnosis, and associate them – for example, 'I understand why you are upset that the treatment has not made the cancer go away'. Some patients might quite reasonably challenge how you can understand if you have not had their experience, but we can all show sympathy if not empathy.

Step 6 S Summary and strategy

- It is important to find out whether the patient is ready to discuss their treatment and plans for their future care.
- Patients who have definite plans tend to be less anxious and uncertain. Patients should be encouraged to share in the treatment planning if they are fit for this. Involving patients in this way also helps them to feel valued, and to feel that their wishes and requests are being valued and noted.

References

1 Baile WF, Buckman R, Lenzi R *et al.* SPIKES – a six-step protocol for delivering bad news: application to the patient with cancer. *Oncologist.* 2000; **5:** 302–11.

Further reading

- Fallowfield L, Jenkins V. Communicating sad, bad and difficult news in medicine. *Lancet.* 2004; **363:** 312–19.
- Lomas D *et al.* The development of best practice in breaking bad news to patients. *Nurs Times.* 2004; **100:** 28–30.

Chapter 4

The angry patient

> I was angry with my friend
> I told my wrath, my wrath did end.
> I was angry with my foe,
> I told it not, my wrath did grow.
>
> William Blake (1757–1827), *Songs of Experience*

Introduction

Anger may not seem to be the most appropriate emotion, and you might not think that this is the time or place for its expression, but anger is a real feeling. The patient is under stress, and it may only be possible to resolve their anger at a later time. They have a lot of free time in hospital for ruminating on their problems and allowing their stress levels to increase! Often the anger is generated by a simple situation which is easily resolved, but inability to deal with that anger, whether it is justified or not, may allow it to grow and become uncontrolled.

C Consider

- Why is the patient angry *now*? What has happened to trigger their anger at this time?
- What is the patient angry about?
- Who are they angry with?
- Is their anger legitimate?
- Is this anger actually an expression of underlying fear?
- Are they angry about a perceived delay in diagnosis?

Reflect on whether you, or other members of the team, picked up cues from relatives which should have been acted upon earlier.

- Did the patient or their relatives express any concerns about lack of involvement in discussion about their treatment or a perceived lack of information?
- Did the relatives make any comment about the patient being distressed or anxious?
- If so, did you make yourself available to deal with these anxieties at the time?
- If there was a reason why you could not address the problem, was this made known to the patient?

A Assess

- How can this problem be effectively addressed?
- Can you deal with the situation now?
- Is there privacy in which to discuss the patient's illness and the reason for their anger? Can anyone else hear what is going on?

If you cannot resolve the problem, who is the best person to deal with the patient's anger and how quickly can they see the patient?

℞ Remedy

It is difficult to deal with anger directed at you when you have been doing your job to the best of your abilities. Even if you recognise that the anger is probably in fact an expression of frustration or fear, it is still difficult to be 'at the receiving end.' Try to be available as soon as possible to hear the problem and resolve it.

- Acknowledge any actual failings or shortcomings, but deal sensitively with any perceived failures in care provision, where in fact the best available care was given.
- Be honest in your replies to criticisms and enquiries.
- Being defensive may not be helpful. It may be perceived as 'having something to hide.'
- Deal with perceived delays in diagnosis by explaining how long it can take for certain diagnostic tests to be completed. Patients and relatives do not know these details. Acknowledge that it might have helped if they had been aware of the expected time it would take for results to be available.

If you are short of time now, try to meet the patient or relatives briefly, making it clear how much time you have available for discussion now and arranging to meet at a mutually agreeable time as soon as possible.

Make sure that there is adequate privacy in which to talk. Anticipate raised voices!

Even if you feel justifiably angry, or an unsubstantiated complaint is made, do not react with anger. Be aware of your body language and try not to let non-verbal cues reveal your true emotions.

Be aware of how you are seen to behave. If you appear very calm and slightly distanced, this can increase the anger of the patient or relatives towards you.

Seek permission to have another member of staff present throughout all discussions. If there is a formal complaint later, you will be glad that you did so. If the patient wishes to have a relative present, too, this is their right. Write up the notes of the discussion promptly and accurately, and have another member of staff present sign them as well.

Do

- Allow the patient or angry relatives to tell you their side of the story first.
- Ask questions to help the patient or relatives to express their anger.
- Let the patient and relatives tell you how they feel.
- Be sympathetic.
- Aim to reach some agreed plan. Depending on the reason for the anger, this may be merely to talk again, or to review the patient's treatment plan, explaining the nature of the hoped for outcome with regard to treatment offered.

Do not

- Start by making defensive or contradictory remarks such as 'It wasn't like that at all'.
- Say things like 'You'll see things differently later when you are feeling better'.
- Ask probing questions in the early stages.

Always

- Give your time now, and listen to any criticism that may be made.
- Offer an explanation or even an apology for any aspect of treatment that has been perceived to be less than optimal.
- Record the discussion with the patient and relatives in the notes, and raise significant issues with the team.

It is important for both the professional carers and the relatives to recognise that it is normal to feel angry about the prospective or actual loss of a loved one, and that anger can sometimes help patients to deal with issues that they find difficult and have been putting off.

Try to develop a joint strategy with the patient and their relatives to help them to cope. Invite the patient and the relatives to tell you when things are getting difficult for them. Sharing their concerns earlier on may help to defuse anger, avoid misunderstandings and help them to cope as the illness progresses.

If there is the possibility of a serious complaint, make notes of this conversation and ask the patient, the relatives and a staff member who was present to sign these later as an accurate record of the discussion. All parties involved have the right to have a copy.

If you fear that a formal complaint may follow, discuss the whole matter honestly and openly with senior colleagues and your professional/defence organisation.

Hopefully the open expression of feelings will clear the air, allowing everyone to move on and to communicate more effectively.

Remember that both the patient and the relatives may need extra support (e.g. Macmillan nurse support or financial advice from a social worker).

Ask the relatives to share any feelings that they have about any aspect of care about which they were unhappy. This approach often defuses anger. It also allows open explanation of simple misunderstandings or previous explanations that were not fully appreciated at a time of extreme stress for the family.

Dealing with anger is exhausting. Even when the anger is directed at you personally, support for the whole team is an absolute necessity.

E Extra information

There are many reasons why patients and relatives become angry. Anger may be directed towards God because of a situation over which they have no control, or may be directed at different people – the team, the patient, the family or even themselves.

The team

Anger may be directed towards members of the team due to the following:

- a perceived lack of accurate or adequate information
- coming to terms with bad news or the changing status of the patient
- misunderstandings about management
- perceived inadequate pain or symptom control in the patient.

The patient

Anger may be directed towards the patient for being ill and leaving the relatives behind.

The family

Anger may be directed towards other family members because of previous or ongoing family problems.

The relatives may:

- feel guilty about not managing the patient at home
- feel that they have no control over the situation.

Complaints from angry patients

It has been noted by the various medical defence bodies that complaints most commonly arise for one of four basic reasons:

- flippancy
- insensitivity
- rudeness
- 'throw-away' remarks.

These are communication problems, not negligence. We all have our bad days, so be on your guard against these simple pitfalls. The patient is having a bad day as well!

Further reading

- Lugton J. *Communicating with Dying People and Their Relatives*. Oxford: Radcliffe Medical Press; 2002.

Chapter 5

Collusion

> Honesty is the first chapter in the book of wisdom
>
> Thomas Jefferson (1743–1826)

Introduction

Collusion is basically an agreement between two parties not to communicate with a third party. In this context, collusion may be between the healthcare professionals and the patient not to inform the family, or between the healthcare professionals and the relatives not to tell the patient something that it is deemed best they should not know.

The basis for such a decision is the desire to protect the third party from anxiety or hurt as a result of being told bad news. However, far from protecting, collusion usually generates problems. Around 80% of 'protected' third parties already know or suspect the truth anyway.

When parties enter into an agreement to collude, a 'cycle of protection' can become established in which the patient seeks to protect the family and the family seeks to protect the patient.

The outcome is almost always unhelpful. A number of things can happen.

- The patient guesses that information is being withheld from them, possibly due to overhearing comments about themselves or having discussions with other patients who seem to be better informed about their illness and treatment options.
- The patient may start to compare their illness and treatment with those of other patients in the hope of finding out about themselves in this way.
- The patient cannot have open discussion with their family or 'let go' emotionally.
- The family may not say goodbye to the patient, and may have difficulties in bereavement.
- The colluders change their behaviour, which arouses suspicion and can generate loss of trust.

C Consider

There are several points about collusion that are worthy of consideration.

- What has motivated the patient or relatives to collude?
- What is the effect on family interactions?
- Think about the rights and needs of the patient. Information is the right of the patient – after all, it is his or her disease. The patient has the right both to have the information and to withhold it from others. He or she may feel the need to protect the family, but there may be serious consequences associated with doing so.

- Think about the needs of the family. They may believe that the patient would not cope with the bad news, and that it will distress him or her. They may be having difficulty in accepting or coming to terms with the news themselves, and be afraid to enter into discussion with the patient.
- The patient or the relatives may feel that if they deny the problem, it will go away.
- There is a risk that failure to communicate may cause isolation, both of the patient and of the family.

A Assess

What does the patient think will happen if the family are aware of his or her disease, treatment options and prognosis?

What do the relatives think will happen if the patient is made aware of his or her diagnosis and prognosis?

Try to assess the current relationship between the patient and his or her family. Are there any obvious difficulties that need to be addressed?

Assess how the patient and their family have coped with difficult situations in the past. Does this give any indication as to how they might cope now, or give any clues as to what support might be needed from the team or other agencies (e.g. Macmillan nursing support or the social worker)?

℞ Remedy

It may be the role of professionals to gently and sensitively dismantle collusion. Honesty is essential, and you need to encourage both the patient and the family to express their feelings, and facilitate more open communication for all.

One or more of the following courses of action may be appropriate.

- Talk with the patient and the family to check their understanding of the current situation.
- Make your responsibility to the patient quite clear. Explain to the relatives that:
  - you will take your cues from the patient with regard to the nature, amount and speed of information sharing with them
  - you will not lie to the patient if he or she should ask what is happening to him or her
  - all of the patient's questions will be answered honestly, and every query will be explored and explained
  - information will be shared sensitively, and not given inappropriately or in a way that will cause avoidable distress.
- Explain that you may involve members of the team who may have a closer relationship than you do with this patient and their family (e.g. another doctor or the social worker).
- Discuss the situation with the multi-professional team and agree a strategy for action.
- If the patient is concerned about disclosure of information to relatives, agree with the patient and do not discuss the situation with the relatives at this

time. Record this in the notes, and let the relatives know why you cannot discuss the patient's situation with them.
- Continue to provide support for both the patient and their family.

The families of patients may find it difficult to discuss these issues, but they may come up in the course of conversation. Be prepared to be called in to help facilitate this discussion.

E Extra information

Collusion is probably the most common communication problem encountered in the early days after the diagnosis of a life-threatening disease. Some families communicate more openly than others, and it may prove impossible to change behaviour that has been present for many years.

A common response is for those who are emotionally close to try to protect each other from further hurt and suffering. In an effort to give the patient a break, well-meaning members of the family may isolate them, thus detaching them from their normal role in the family and inadvertently removing much of the activity that gave meaning to the patient's life.

Bringing a family member or friend into the bad news interview carries the risk that the information has been heard by a third party and will be shared among the wider circle of family or friends. This may not be the case, but it is hard to assess what will happen after the patient leaves the consulting room.

'Family' may mean more than blood relatives of the patient. It is important to recognise that biological links may not be the most important ones, and there may be a 'significant other', a person who is not a blood relative of the patient but who is seen as more important to them. This can be difficult for blood relatives to accept, but the patient's wishes must be respected.

The patient may cope by denying the illness (see below). Denial should be suspected if there is failure to comply with the doctor's advice or to plan realistically.

Sometimes the patient's imaginings can be worse than the actual diagnosis. This can lead to fears and anxieties that are unfounded, and these can often be resolved by knowing the truth.

You will have been effective if the patient and their significant others feel well supported, and you still have a good dialogue with them without compromising your relationship with the patient.

Over time, the collusion may change. You can then explore how well the patient and the family are coping, and offer appropriate input.

Further reading

- Surbone A, Zwitter M, editors. Communication with the cancer patient: information and truth. *Ann N Y Acad Sci*. 1997; **809**. (This entire volume deals with acceptable methods of communication, sharing and withholding of information in various cultures and countries.)

Chapter 6

Confidentiality

> This is a free country, madam. We have a right to share your privacy in a public place.
>
> Sir Peter Ustinov (1956) in *Romanoff and Juliet*

Introduction

Absolute confidentiality is almost impossible to achieve. We can do our best to minimise unintentional information leakage in telephone conversations and face-to-face communication, but a curtain round a bed is no sound barrier, and we do depend on other patients and relatives not to eavesdrop, and to respect the privacy of others.

The case notes can be openly viewed by many healthcare professionals, and email, faxing and other modern communication methods are not secure.

One of the authors, attending hospital as a patient, had a full view of a set of investigation results that had been left beside a hand-washing station at the entrance to the ward. The person who left the notes there may have been reducing the risk of spreading MRSA, but did nothing for the privacy of the patient concerned!

Added to this, patients probably share information with significant others, and they have no control over who those individuals tell.

C Consider

How much confidentiality does the patient expect or want? Are they happy for relevant entries to be made in their notes and do they realise who will be able to see the notes?

Is the patient aware that their refusal to have information recorded in their notes could result in delays in effective management being offered?

Is the patient aware that certain disclosures are normally made to other members of the team in order to plan best care, and that they may be included in audits or research, albeit anonymously?

There is also a small possibility that you might be legally obliged to release information to a third party.

A Assess

Is the patient competent to make decisions about disclosure or non-recording of information? Are they fully aware of the possible outcomes of their decision?

What are the possible outcomes of information not being shared with the multi-professional team that is caring for the patient?

What is the risk of information being seen by individuals other than those who were intended to see it? Does your department use email or fax to speed referrals? If so, can you be sure that these are as secure and confidential as the patient would wish?

℞ Remedy

Agree with the patient what will be recorded in their notes, who can see the notes and what methods can be used for sharing information with other professionals. Make the patient aware of the possibility of delay if the medium used for sharing information is significantly slower than that normally used (e.g. a letter sent by post compared with an emailed or faxed referral).

E Extra information

If there is doubt about the diagnosis, if the illness is due to an industrial disease or if a post-mortem may be required for another reason, there may be a duty incumbent upon the doctor to make the results known in the interests of the public. It may be relevant to discuss this difficult subject with the patient and their family.

Further guidance on this subject can be downloaded from the General Medical Council website (www.gmc-uk.org) or may be obtained from the General Medical Council by requesting the booklets *Confidentiality: protecting and providing information*[1] and *Confidentiality: protecting and providing information (2004) – 'frequently asked questions'*.[2]

References

1 General Medical Council. *Confidentiality: protecting and providing information*. London: General Medical Council; 2004. (Available from General Medical Council, 178 Great Portland Street, London W1W 5JE.)

2 General Medical Council. *Confidentiality: protecting and providing information (2004) – frequently asked questions*. London: General Medical Council; 2004. (Available from General Medical Council, 178 Great Portland Street, London W1W 5JE.)

Further reading

- Dein S, Thomas K. To tell or not to tell. *Eur J Palliat Care*. 2002; **9**: 209–12. (This paper looks at cultural and religious practices relating to communicating a fatal prognosis.)

Chapter 7

Denial

> The art of living is the art of knowing how to believe lies.
>
> Cesare Pavese

Introduction

Denial is a primitive defence mechanism that enables individuals to cope with very distressing events or thoughts.

We shall consider three types of denial:

1 'healthy denial'
2 'unhealthy denial'
3 'no further attention denial'.

Healthy denial

'Healthy denial' helps the person to adjust and become accustomed to a major loss before responding to the painful reality of the situation (e.g. accepting the fact that they have cancer). Healthy denial:

- allows the person to manage unwelcome situations they cannot change (e.g. denying that they are losing weight as disease advances by buying smaller clothes)
- gives the person time to become accustomed to the facts before responding to the pain of the situation
- helps the person to adjust to ideas that cause them distress (e.g. 'I'll beat this cancer yet').

The initial response of denial is likely to be temporary or only part of a continually changing picture. Sometimes the patient will seem to know and accept the reality of their situation, while at other times they will speak and behave as if nothing is wrong.

Unhealthy denial

'Unhealthy denial' is a reaction that creates a barrier and prevents the person from adjusting to a new situation. Clues to unhealthy denial include the following:

- evidence that the patient is not coping
- isolation from family and friends
- risk of endangering the patient's best interests or treatment.

No further attention denial

'No further attention denial' is our preferred term to describe those few patients who simply will not discuss their illness, but who attend all appointments and comply fully with all treatments. They prepare for their future, make the necessary arrangements for their funeral, and thereafter ignore their illness and refuse to discuss it. In other words, they deal with the issues promptly and efficiently, ignoring them thereafter. It is an unusual situation and very difficult to deal with.

In a sense this denial (if it is indeed denial) is healthy but, since any form of discussion is virtually impossible, one can never be confident that it was managed well.

C Consider

What type of denial is the patient showing?

Can you, by 'putting yourself in their shoes', decide what feelings and issues the person is avoiding? We accept that this is virtually impossible to do, but it is probably the best attempt we can make to see the situation from the patient's perspective.

A Assess

Do you know for how long this denial has been going on? Who else has observed it? What is the impact of this denial on the patient and their family?

Ask the multi-professional team about it.

- Do they all feel that it is denial?
- How are other team members responding to this situation?
- Is there a coordinated plan to deal with the denial?

Assess the nature of the denial. Explore the issues that the patient is avoiding, and decide who is the best team member to talk to the patient and their relatives.

℞ Remedy

Reassess the patient's physical status. Pain and other symptoms may be interfering with their emotional state. Have you talked with the relatives recently?

Devise your plan of action as a team.

Determine which professional has the closest relationship with the patient, and invite them to have a discussion with the patient. Decide which of the following courses of action may be appropriate.

- If denial is healthy, there may be no need for intervention, reinforcement or confrontation. To be effective, you need to plan carefully. You also need to understand and accept the feelings that emerge.
- If denial is unhealthy, you need to explore how to help the individual to come to terms with the situation. This may include confronting their denial, which can be difficult and may cause problems between patient and carer. Sometimes it may be better to leave things for now, be aware of the problem and look for an opportunity to deal with it at a later date.

Record the outcome and inform colleagues so that the team knows how best to respond.

E Extra information

Bearing in mind that denial has a protective function, being part of a team looking after a patient in denial can be a stressful experience, and you may feel that, initially, it might be easier to have less-open conversations.

There may also be differences of opinion within the team, or pressure from relatives to force the patient to accept what is happening. If you don't have a coordinated plan, you could all be responding to the patient and the relatives in different ways, which could cause more problems. The patient may already have had a dialogue with another professional who might be the most appropriate person for them to speak to.

Continued denial is inappropriate when someone vulnerable is dependent upon the patient, such as a young child, an elderly person, or someone with physical or mental health problems, including learning disability.

Denial should not be reinforced or unnecessarily confronted by your intervention. It is important that the patient comes to terms with the illness in their own way. Rarely, reinforcement has a useful role – for example, when it is obvious that the patient's death is imminent, yet they firmly believe that their health is improving. It may be unrealistic to expect them to face death totally unprepared.

Further reading

- Dein S. Working with the patient who is in denial. *Eur J Palliat Care*. 2005; **12:** 251–3.
- Wilkinson S, Fellowes D, Leliopoulou C. Does truth-telling influence patients' psychological distress? *Eur J Palliat Care*. 2005; **12:** 124–6.

Chapter 8

Distancing oneself from the patient

'Sorry, I didn't see you there.'
'That's all right', said Eeyore. 'No one ever does.'

AA Milne

Introduction

We all occasionally meet patients from whom we keep a distance for one reason or another. Ask yourself what it is about you, or your past experience, that makes it difficult for you to interact with this patient.

C Consider

What is your usual 'distance' from patients? You must find your own comfortable distance. This will be different for different patients and for individual carers.

Ask other members of the team if they are having difficulty relating to this patient. There are some patients to whom we cannot get 'close' for many reasons.

A Assess

Think about possible reasons why you are distancing yourself from the patient.

- Is it because of a communication difficulty? This may be because you are unable to relate to each other, or it may be due to an accent, a different first language or a physical disability causing speech problems.
- Is it because you can relate to their illness, perhaps because a person close to you died from a similar illness? If this is bringing back painful memories, it may be best for you to ask another team member to take over the care of the patient. You are not 'weak' for asking for such help. It is natural, and if either your judgement or your ability to remain objective are being affected, ask for help.
- Is it due to fear that the patient may start crying or shouting at you?
- Is it due to fear that you will not be able to answer difficult questions?

Distancing may be an early indicator of 'burnout'. Could this be the reason? If so, try to set up adequate support systems and supervision outside of the working environment to help to offset this.

℞ Remedy

Acknowledge that there is a problem with a particular patient, and take the remedial actions appropriate to the self-assessment you have conducted. Ensure that your actions/feelings do not generalise to other patients.

Make sure that you are receiving adequate support from members of the team, and invite another member of the team to take over for a while.

Ensure that you have adequate rest and time for relaxation.
Having taken these actions:

- check whether you find yourself more able to make contact with this particular patient. Has the original difficulty been resolved?
- check whether you feel better supported by members of the team
- remember that distancing oneself is a coping mechanism, and may be a sign of excessive stress.

If the patient is having difficulty in communicating due to a physical problem, seek appropriate help for them. If possible, seek the help of a nurse specialist or other colleague with experience of working with patients with sensory impairment.

E Extra information

Often distancing results from communication difficulty, sometimes related to a sensory impairment or learning disability.

Sensory impairment is physical. As has often been said, 'deaf is not daft'. The patient is not necessarily disabled in terms of their mental function. Do not ask a third party to answer on the patient's behalf.

If you ask relatives to use sign language for a deaf person, you have no control over how they interpret or amend your question or the patient's response. It is reasonable to ask them not to reword or interpret questions or answers, and to seek clarification if they are unsure what you are asking. Simplify your questions to avoid the need for rewording.

Written text is easier to read if it is printed using black ink on pale pastel-coloured paper rather than bright white paper. Use a reasonable size of letters (slightly larger than this typeface, e.g. a size 14 font), and avoid using upper-case letters throughout the text. Dyslexic patients might find the 'Arial' font on a computer or word processor easier to read.

Further reading

No journal papers on this topic were identified.

Chapter 9

Getting too close to the patient

> Have no friends not equal to yourself.
>
> Confucius

Introduction

We all have patients to whom we become emotionally close, but the risk of emotional burnout then becomes a real possibility.

C Consider

What is your actual role in the multi-professional team? Do you need to be so involved, or can you reduce your input without compromising patient care?

A Assess

Is it just you, or are other members of the team also becoming 'too involved'? Does this patient need a lot of input and is this hard to achieve without getting too close?

Review your relationship with this particular patient and their family. Whose dependency need is being fulfilled through this relationship?

How much of this 'attachment' is felt just by you and how much is felt by the patient? How might the patient react to the suggestion that you might reduce your input or invite a colleague to take over some of your role?

℞ Remedy

Discuss the situation with a colleague or within the team if that is more appropriate. If the problem is the patient's dependency on you, then it is a matter for the team to resolve together.

Decide who might be the best person in your team to assume the role of 'key worker.'

Continue to do your normal work, but with assistance from colleagues, reducing your contact with the patient and their family. Don't overstep the agreed new boundaries.

If necessary, take advice from colleagues about whether the situation ought to be discussed with the patient and/or the family.

Remain sensitive to the patient's vulnerability, and try to avoid provoking any sense of guilt, awkwardness or isolation. This may involve introducing other team members to the patient, being less involved in discussion about the patient, and supporting the building of trust between the patient and other team members.

E Extra information

There is a saying, by an unknown person, that 'empathy is your pain in my heart'. If you have been feeling the patient's pain, you need to review how you are coping with distancing yourself appropriately from the patient to whom you became too close.

On a weekly basis, or more often if appropriate, ask yourself the following questions:

- am I less overwhelmed by my involvement?
- have I formed a different but no less supportive relationship with the patient?
- is the patient receiving adequate support from others?
- is the support I am receiving from colleagues meeting my needs? If not, do I need to seek professional help or counselling?

Further reading

No journal papers on this topic were identified.

Chapter 10

The patient who refuses to talk

Still-born Silence, thou that art
Floodgate of the deeper heart.

Richard Flecknoe (Irish priest and poet, died *c.*1678), *Invocation of Silence*

Introduction

Occasionally, one comes across a patient who refuses to discuss their illness in any way. They may discuss all other topics, but the subject of their illness is greeted with silence and refusal to enter into any discussion. Patients may also show a definite disapproval of any discussion taking place with their relatives or carers, and this creates a difficulty, as one could commit an act of assault by enforcing any examination or treatment without consent.

C Consider

Does the reason for not talking appear to be personal, psychological or physical?

A Assess

Is the patient still able to talk? Has a new problem developed that makes speech difficult or impossible?

Has there been a change in the patient's circumstances? For example, do they appear to be:

- confused
- depressed
- exhausted and unable to be bothered talking
- in pain?

Is there any suggestion of a neurological problem that is preventing speech? Assess the non-verbal cues.

If you have been distancing yourself, either because you are having difficulty dealing with this patient or because you were getting too close to them, is the patient aware of this and refusing to talk because they see this as the most appropriate way of dealing with the changing relationship?

Does the patient think that you do not have enough time to talk to them?

Is the patient too embarrassed to discuss their problem? Perhaps they disclosed something that they now feel they should have kept to themselves, or they are anxious about it being recorded in their notes.

Ask the other members of the team if the patient is not talking to them either.

Remember that if a patient stops talking, it is not necessarily a criticism of you. It may simply relate to how they feel and their understanding of their illness.

However, even if they don't wish to talk, you should continue to listen. Do not fall into the traps of:

- probing for information
- providing advice
- responding with your advice and suggestions.

The patient will speak to you when they are ready. Just be there ready to listen and respond to them.

℞ Remedy

Having assessed the reasons for this failure to communicate, give a clear explanation to the family. Do not let the relatives feel that the patient is being ignored or that their concerns are not recognised.

Continue your relationship with the patient and do not ignore them. Visit regularly to offer them adequate opportunities to speak to you.

Involve another member of staff with whom they might communicate.

Maintain your contact with the family and try to gain insight into how the family functions, as this may have some bearing on what is going on.

Appraise the team and try to develop a coordinated plan of management for the patient and their family.

E Extra information

The patient's refusal to talk is not necessarily a reflection on your care, but they may still be giving you a message.

They may be saying 'I'm really angry' – with God, you and the team, themselves, or simply because they have cancer and cannot cope with what is going on and don't wish to think about it or talk about it. This may be a form of denial, and it may be their only perceived coping mechanism.

Part 2

Therapy review

Chapter 11

A brief review of how drugs work

> Imperative drugging – the ordering of medicine in any and every malady – is no longer regarded as the chief function of the doctor.
> Sir William Osler (1849–1919) *Aequanimitas, with other addresses*

Introduction

This chapter deals only with the most basic issues of pharmacology relevant to cancer care, and some useful books are listed in the Further reading section.

Cancer patients are likely to have a number of symptoms and may be taking several different medications. The risk of interactions increases with the number of medications prescribed, so a basic understanding of pharmacology is helpful. Compliance with medication tends to be worse when several drugs are prescribed, so this may be worth considering, and it may be possible to use one drug to achieve control of more than one symptom. An example of this would be the use of cimetidine both to control malignant sweating and for gastric protection.

Medications are usually administered by mouth, by injection or by transdermal absorption. What happens next?

There are several ways in which the drug may act:

- action via a receptor
- action via a second messenger
- action via an indirect alteration of the effects of an endogenous agonist
- inhibition of transport processes
- enzyme inhibition
- action by other methods.

Action via a receptor

A receptor is a specific protein, located either in the cell membrane or within the cell itself. For each specific receptor, there is a specific group of drugs or substances (ligands) that specifically bind to that receptor to produce a pharmacological effect. Three types of ligands exist:

- agonists
- antagonists
- partial agonists.

Agonists are ligands that bind to a receptor to produce a response. Adrenaline is an agonist. It binds to a specific ß-adrenoreceptor in the heart and causes tachycardia. The more receptors the agonist binds to, the greater its effect. Interestingly, the word 'agonist' originally described athletes and athletic combatants.

Antagonists are ligands that prevent an agonist from binding to a receptor, thereby preventing its effect. A common example is propranolol, which is a ß-receptor antagonist (or beta-blocker).

Partial agonists, in contrast to agonists, cannot produce a full effect even when bound to the maximum number of receptors available. As a result, above a certain level, increasing the amount of the partial agonist available has no additional pharmacological effect. This is called the 'ceiling effect'.

Partial agonists may affect the action of other agonists and thus appear to act as antagonists. This mixed action is known as *partial antagonism.*

Receptor subtypes

Some receptors have subtypes, and this allows selectivity in the action of the ligands. For example, there are at least two types of beta-blocker receptors – the $ß_1$ type, which is found in the heart, and the $ß_2$ type, which is found in the lung. Propranolol acts on both, whereas atenolol is more selective, acting only on the $ß_1$-receptors.

The effects of long-term use of drugs must also be considered, because with long-term administration, *adaptive responses* may occur. These are usually accompanied by either an increase ('up-regulation') or a decrease ('down-regulation') in the numbers of receptors in the tissues. The resultant changes may be responsible for either beneficial or adverse effects of the drugs involved. For example:

- *slow onset of action.* Antidepressants may cause changes in the receptors in the brain, but it takes a few weeks before the full response to treatment is seen
- *withdrawal syndromes.* Long-term changes may become unopposed when the drug is withdrawn. This may be seen after the prolonged use of benzodiazepines for chronic anxiety, when the changes that have occurred in the receptors may remain unopposed. A similar situation can occur after long-term *abuse* of opioids. However, it is not a feature when opioids are used correctly for long-term control of pain, and patients should be reassured that long-term use of opioids is safe when they are correctly prescribed.

Action via a second messenger

Agonists produce their effects in one of two ways – via another chemical in the cell (sometimes called the 'second messenger'), or by altering the activity of an ion channel linked to the receptor.

Action via an indirect alteration of the effects of an endogenous agonist

Antagonists can produce their effects by directly or indirectly opposing the action of an endogenous agonist.

Physiological antagonism describes the effect of drugs that have a physiological effect which is opposite to that of other drugs. For example, glucagon is a physiological antagonist of insulin.

Increased endogenous release describes the situation where the action of an endogenous agonist is enhanced by the drug. For example, amphetamines stimulate increased release of dopamine from nerve endings.

Inhibition of endogenous reuptake. Some drugs produce their effects by preventing reuptake of an endogenous agonist, and thereby enhancing its effects. Many antidepressants work in this way by inhibiting reuptake of neurotransmitters such as noradrenaline.

Inhibition of endogenous metabolism. If a drug inhibits the metabolism of an endogenous agonist, it will enhance its effects. Vigabatrin inhibits γ-aminobutyric acid (GABA) metabolism, thereby suppressing seizures.

Prevention of endogenous release of agonists reduces effects. For example, the angiotensin-converting enzyme (ACE) inhibitors block the formation of angiotensin II, which blocks the endogenous release of aldosterone, which in turn results in retention of potassium.

Inhibition of transport processes

Inhibition of transport processes is important because various cations, including calcium, sodium and potassium, and other substances, such as organic acids in the kidneys, are important for maintaining normal cell function. Many diuretics act by inhibiting sodium reabsorption (e.g. furosemide). Calcium antagonists selectively inhibit transport of calcium across cell membranes. Potassium movement stabilises cell membranes, and cellular activity is reduced by opening the potassium channels and increased by closing them. Smooth muscle relaxants such as minoxidil open the potassium channels and reduce blood pressure, while sulphonylureas close the potassium channels and result in increased release of insulin.

Enzyme inhibition

Enzyme inhibition works in several ways, depending on the normal action of the enzyme. Relevant examples include allopurinol, an inhibitor of xanthine oxidase, which normally converts the very water-soluble xanthine and hypoxanthine to much less-soluble uric acid. They are more rapidly excreted in their water-soluble state.

Monoamine oxidase inhibitors (MAOIs) produce an antidepressant effect by inhibiting the metabolism of the monoamines 5-hydroxytryptamine (5HT), noradrenaline (norepinephrine) and dopamine in the brain.

Enzyme activation of plasminogen is the mode of action of several thrombolytic agents, and factor VIII acts by replacing deficient enzymes in the clotting pathway.

Action by other methods

This includes the mode of action of the chelating agents, which can be used to speed up the removal of metals from the body. Examples include EDTA, which chelates many divalent and trivalent metals, desferrioxamine for iron, and penicillamine for copper.

Mannitol is an osmotic diuretic that is freely filtered by the glomerulus but poorly reabsorbed by the renal tubules. By increasing the concentration of osmotically active particles in the tubular fluid, it draws in water and increases the urinary volume.

Analgesics act in a variety of ways which can be summarised as follows:

- altering emotional responses (e.g. anxiolytics and tricyclics)
- altering spinal cord modulation (e.g. opioids, nitrous oxide)
- interrupting transmission along the peripheral nerve (e.g. local anaesthetics)

- reducing peripheral nerve excitation (e.g. non-steroidal anti-inflammatory drugs (NSAIDs) and corticosteroids)
- suppressing abnormal neuronal activity (e.g. anticonvulsants, mexiletine).

Adverse drug reactions and interactions

One of the common fears expressed by patients is that of having an adverse drug reaction, and patients often ask 'What are the side-effects of this medicine?'

In this chapter we shall look at the broad issues relating to adverse drug reactions (ADRs) and adverse drug interactions (ADIs).

Drugs that either block or stimulate receptors, use carrier molecules to bind to various sites, block channels or depend on enzyme activation will act on all of the sites in the body, not just those of the diseased organ. The adverse event may thus be predictable, even with the newer, more 'selective' drugs.

Some of the commoner ADRs include those of NSAIDs, which can exacerbate asthma or cause peptic ulceration due to their effect on prostaglandin synthesis, and those of tricyclic drugs which, due to their antimuscarinic effects, cause a dry mouth.

Many ADRs can be avoided by judicious prescribing, but the risk of ADIs increases with the number of drugs prescribed, and polypharmacy is relatively common in cancer care.

Interactions may be divided into six broad categories as follows:

- interactions that occur during drug absorption
- interactions that occur during drug distribution
- interactions that occur during drug metabolism
- interactions that occur between drugs at their site of action
- interactions that occur because of plasma half-life mismatch
- interactions that occur because of additive or antagonistic effects of two drugs.

For more detailed information, the reader should consult the *British National Formulary (BNF)*, Appendix 1.

Interactions that occur during drug absorption

Antacids containing aluminium, calcium and magnesium cause impaired absorption of several drugs and may interfere with enteric coatings. Examples include ACE inhibitors, antibiotics, anti-epileptic drugs, antifungal drugs, bisphosphonates and some H_2-blockers.

Interactions that occur during drug distribution

Many drugs bind loosely to plasma proteins or tissue proteins during distribution to the site of action. When two or more drugs compete for the same protein-binding sites, one may displace the other, releasing it as an active drug in the plasma. This may result in the released drug reaching toxic levels.

Interactions that occur during drug metabolism

Most drugs are metabolised in the liver by the cytochrome P_{450} oxidase enzyme system. This usually renders the drug less active and prepares it for excretion via the kidneys. Several drugs inhibit the cytochrome P_{450} oxidase enzyme system, allowing the drug to build up in the plasma, and other drugs induce the cytochrome P_{450} oxidase enzymes, resulting in more rapid elimination and failure to produce the desired therapeutic effect. Three examples are listed below.

- Cimetidine, by acting as an enzyme inhibitor, increases the effects of at least 17 different drug classes, including antibiotics, anticonvulsants, beta-blockers, fluorouracil, NSAIDs and pethidine.
- Allopurinol interacts with ciclosporin.
- The imidazole antifungals interfere with several other drugs, including corticosteroids.

Interactions that occur between drugs at their site of action

These interactions occur when two drugs compete for binding sites at the same receptor, enzyme or carrier channel. The most common example is that of the $ß_1$-blockers, which diminish the effects of anti-asthmatic $ß_2$-agonists.

Interactions that occur because of plasma half-life mismatch

The most relevant example in cancer care is the use of naloxone to reverse the effect of another opioid, such as diamorphine. This should not be necessary if the drugs have been prescribed correctly, but it may occasionally be required. Naloxone displaces morphine and diamorphine from the opioid μ-receptors, rapidly reversing opioid toxicity. The problem is that the half-life of naloxone is 30–60 minutes, whereas that of diamorphine is 3–4 hours. When the naloxone has been eliminated, the circulating diamorphine reoccupies the opioid receptors, and the symptoms and signs of toxicity may recur.

Interactions that occur because of additive or antagonistic effects of two drugs

The additive effects of two drugs can be used to good effect, as is the case with many commercially marketed combined preparations. On the other hand, some combinations are potentially dangerous – for example, ACE inhibitors and NSAIDs, which both reduce secretion of aldosterone and can result in dangerous hyperkalaemia.

Further reading

- British Medical Association and Royal Pharmaceutical Society of Great Britain. Appendix 1: Interactions. In: *British National Formulary 52*. London: British Medical Association and Royal Pharmaceutical Society of Great Britain; 2006.
- McGavock H. *How Drugs Work*. Oxford: Radcliffe Medical Press; 2003.
- Twycross R, Wilcock A, Charlesworth S *et al*. *PCF2 Palliative Care Formulary*. Oxford: Radcliffe Medical Press; 2002.

Chapter 12

Complementary therapies

> As to diseases, make a habit of two things – to help, or at least, to do no harm.
>
> Hippocrates (Greek physician, *c*.460 BC – *c*.377 BC), *Epidemics, Book* 1

Introduction

The words 'complementary' and 'alternative' are sometimes used by patients to mean one and the same thing. In this text, we shall use them as described below.

Alternative cancer treatments are those that claim to prolong the patient's life, to reduce the symptoms caused by the burden of tumour, and to be a replacement for conventional medicines.

Complementary therapies are used alongside conventional ones, and usually do not claim to replace them by providing a cure. Individual practitioners may make claims which suggest that complementary therapies can offer more than this definition suggests.

Attempts to integrate complementary and alternative medicine (CAM) into the NHS are continuing. At the time of writing, the Foundation for Integrated Health is setting up an Integrated Health Association with the remit of supporting delivery of integrated care throughout the UK.

The Medicines and Healthcare products Regulatory Agency (MHRA) is regulating homoeopathic and herbal medicines.

In May 2006, the Complementary and Alternative Medicine Specialist Library was launched to provide healthcare professionals and the public with the best available evidence for CAM. This is part of the National Library for Health, and up-to-date information will be available on its website (www.library.nhs.uk/cam).

C Consider

It is estimated that about 20% of the population use complementary or alternative medicine of some sort. There may be several perfectly good reasons for this, but it might be worth exploring the reasons why your patient wishes to consider these options now.

- Are they disillusioned in some way with the orthodox medicine and healthcare provision?
- Is it about the time spent with the patient? An average appointment with the GP lasts 10 minutes; an appointment with a homoeopath could last almost ten times as long.
- Is it about the patient having control and choice or responsibility for their health and treatment?

Patients cite a number of reasons for wishing to try CAM, including the following:

- availability without long waiting lists
- control – attending only as often as the patient wishes
- holistic concept
- low-tech, high-touch appeal
- non-invasive treatment
- perceived effectiveness
- perceived safety
- time spent in consultations
- individualised treatment.

However, these are the 'positive' reasons that a patient might readily offer. They might not so readily admit to doubts and 'negative' thoughts, including the following:

- desperation to try everything, whatever it costs
- dissatisfaction with the treatment offered or the staff offering the treatment
- false belief and hope that CAM can provide a cure which is not available in orthodox medicine
- issues concerning modern science and technology (including ADRs and testing drugs on animals)
- recognition that orthodox treatment is not helping, but reluctance to accept this, accompanied by a desire to try something else.

You also need to think about the following issues:

- contraindications to the complementary therapy must be considered and addressed
- cost must be considered. Some therapies are not available on the NHS. The cost-benefit ratio may be harder to quantify!
- does starting a planned complementary or alternative treatment involve stopping a clearly beneficial conventional treatment?
- is the treatment evidence based? Most complementary medicine is under-researched
- are there any reported risks or side-effects?
- what is the value of the therapy? Has this been validated in a reputable journal after a suitably conducted clinical trial?
- is there any written information from reputable sources? Is there any information for the patient?

A Assess

You need to consider whether the patient's wish to use complementary therapy is just a way of expressing their need for any of the following:

- clearer communication and time to discuss their symptoms
- explanation and reassurance that you and the team have no objection to them trying a complementary therapy in addition to the treatments they are already receiving
- the opportunity to explore why other treatment options have not been offered. Patients with the same basic diagnoses (e.g. 'lung cancer') do wonder why their treatment schedules differ, and may question why they are not

being offered something that another patient (with a different histology) is receiving.

Discuss the current orthodox treatment with both the patient and the family. Do they have any unfulfilled hopes? Is there any misunderstanding that needs to be addressed or corrected?

Find out how the patient views the complementary therapy that they wish to try. Do they have any incorrect or unfounded hopes about the outcome of the treatment?

℞ Remedy

Since neither of the authors has training or expertise in CAM, we shall provide only a very brief review of some of the more popular therapies, and we have included details of sources from which further information may be obtained.

We have noted that very little good-quality research has been undertaken, and an evidence base for these therapies has not been found in any of the journals devoted to evidence-based practice. This is because most of these therapies have developed outside the scientific and research-based therapies. It is also argued by those who practise CAM that if patients feel better, they do not need to know about the 'evidence.'

There are a few basic principles that can still be applied, whatever our knowledge and views.

It is important to reinforce the fact that adopting a complementary treatment need not cut the patient off from conventional therapies, and that the conventional treatment must continue exactly as prescribed.

Advise patients that at present only osteopathy and chiropractic are regulated by law.

Patients should therefore:

- ask their doctor about the safety and advisability of CAM for them
- be aware that CAM practitioners often do not communicate with the GP or hospital doctor, and vice versa, so the patient's medical history is not shared
- contact the relevant professional membership organisation and obtain as much information as possible
- only see a registered CAM practitioner.

After the patient has attended a complementary therapist, ask them whether it was helpful and in what ways they feel that the therapy improved their quality of life and their perception of their current state of health.

Acupuncture

Acupuncture, which uses fine needles inserted at specific points in the body, has been used for thousands of years in China and other eastern countries. It has been shown to be effective for a number of conditions.

Further information

British Acupuncture Council
Tel: 0208 735 0400
Website: www.acupuncture.org.uk

Alexander technique

This is about posture, movement and dealing with tension and how it relates to the underlying cause. It is taught to patients who then continue the practice at home.

Further information

Society of Teachers of the Alexander Technique
Tel: 0845 230 7828
Website: www.stat.org.uk (provides details of teachers near your workplace)

Aromatherapy

Aromatherapy uses healing plant oils and massage. Patients may be confused and think that the oils used by therapists are identical to the very diluted ones which are available very cheaply in high street shops. This is not the case, and patients need to be carefully selected for aromatherapy, as certain oils cannot be used in particular medical conditions.

Further information

International Federation of Professional Aromatherapists
Tel: 01455 637 987
Website: www.ifparoma.org
Email: admin@IFPAroma.org

Chinese herbal medicine

A mixture of traditional formulas and tinctures is used, many dating back to 3500 BC. Adverse reactions, contamination with heavy metals and interactions with orthodox medicines have all been reported. There is no regulation of this therapy, and an unqualified person can set up the service.

Further information

There is no statutory regulatory body, but a register of qualified Chinese herbal practitioners can be found at www.rchm.co.uk.

Chiropractic

This technique specialises in the disorders of the nervous system and spinal column. The Medical Research Council has demonstrated that the technique is effective for back pain.

Further information

British Chiropractic Association
Tel: 0118 950 5950
Website: www.chiropractic-uk.co.uk

Crystal therapy

Crystals are used to absorb, diffuse, direct and focus energy within the body, encouraging natural healing and restoring biorhythms.

Further information

Information, and a list of healers, may be obtained from www.crystaltherapy.co.uk.

Herbal remedies

As with Chinese herbal medicine, there can be many impurities in herbal medicines and they are not regulated. There is great potential for interaction with prescribed medicines, and no way of checking the precise formulation of the product, as ingredients may be altered or exchanged and may be misleadingly documented on the packaging. Allergic reactions, drug interactions and toxic reactions have all been reported.

Further information

No reliable source has been identified.

Homeopathy

This is a holistic system of healing based on the principle that 'like heals like'.

Patients are given very highly diluted medicines. Opinions vary widely about the effectiveness of homeopathy, and the 'evidence' is lacking, but many patients report benefit.[1]

Further information

Faculty of Homoeopaths
Tel: 0870 444 3950
Website: www.trusthomeopathy.org
(Please note the variation in spelling of the word 'homeopathy.' The website address is spelled as given above, even though the alternative spelling, 'homoeopathy', is used in their letterhead.)

Massage

No research evidence was found, but this cannot be claimed as a cure for cancer. So long as patients recognise this, there is no reason not to attend for massage if it makes the patient feel better and helps them to relax.

Further information

General Council for Massage Therapy
Tel: 0870 850 4452
Website: www.gcmt.org.uk

Osteopathy

This therapy involves manipulation for a range of musculoskeletal problems involving bone, joints and connective tissues. No information was found about the use of osteopathy in cancer.

Further information

British Osteopathic Council
Tel: 0207 357 6655
Website: www.osteopathy.org.uk

Reflexology

Reflexology is a system based on the belief that reflex points situated on the feet act as nerve receptors for the whole body.

Further information

Association of Reflexologists
Tel: 0870 567 3320
Website: www.aor.org.uk

Reiki

Reiki is a Japanese system of laying on of hands in a carefully controlled sequence. It is claimed to control and heal pain.

Further information

The Reiki Association can provide further information and a list of practitioners, and can be accessed at www.reikiassociation.org.uk.

Spiritual healing

Spiritual healing claims to channel energy to re-energise the patient to deal with their illness.

Further information

National Federation of Spiritual Healers
Tel: 0845 123 2777
Website: www.nfsh.org.uk

E Extra information

The link between all of the complementary therapies is that they all highlight the individuality of the person and the power of the body to heal itself. Zoning in on the concept of homeostasis, it makes sense to treat the whole body or whole person, and this is a central theme for most of the therapies.

We list here some organisations that might be of assistance to you.

Bristol Cancer Help Centre

Tel: 0117 9809 500. Office hours 09.30am – 5.00pm Monday to Friday
Helpline: 0845 1232 310

Website: www.bristolcancerhelp.org
Email: helpline@bristolcancerhelp.org

British Complementary Medicine Association

Tel: 0845 3345 5977. Office hours 10.00am – 4.30pm Monday to Friday
Website: www.bcma.co.uk
Email: info@bcma.org

Complementary Cancer Care Trust

Tel: 01322 493 344. Office hours 10.00am – 4.00pm Monday to Friday
Website: www.ccctrust.org.uk
Email: enquiries@ccctrust.org.uk

Institute for Complementary Medicine

Tel: 020 7237 5165. Office hours 10.00am – 3.30pm Monday to Friday
Website: www.i-c-m.org.uk
Email: info@i-c-m.org.uk

Complementary and Alternative Medicine Specialist Library

Website: www.library.nhs.uk/cam
This service provides healthcare professionals and the public with the best available evidence for complementary and alternative medicine.

References

1 Ernst E, Hyland M, Stevens P. Is homeopathy good for anything? *Science Public Affairs*. 2005; **December issue:** 20–21.

Further reading

- Baum M. Paying a complement: should the NHS fund alternative medicine? *New Generalist*. 2006; **4:** 26–7. (This paper forms part of *The Complementary and Alternative Medicine Debate: is existing evidence enough to justify NHS funding?* The reference by Lewith listed below provides an alternative viewpoint in the same debate.)
- Dean ME. 'An innocent deception': placebo controls in the St Petersburg homoeopathy trial, 1829–1830. *J R Soc Med*. 2006; **99:** 375–6.
- Ernst E. *Complementary Medicine: an objective appraisal*. Oxford: Butterworth-Heinemann; 1996.
- Ernst E. The 'Smallwood Report': method or madness. *Br J Gen Pract*. 2006; **56:** 64–5.
- Jeffries D. Homeopathy – a benign deception? *Br J Gen Pract*. 2005; **55:** 490.
- Kelly J. Toxicity and adverse effects of herbal complementary therapy. *Prof Nurse*. 2002; **17:** 562–5.
- Lewith G. The complementary and alternative medicine debate: is existing evidence enough to justify NHS funding? *New Generalist*. 2006; **4:** 28–9.
- Lomas C. Building the case for CAM. *Nurs Times*. 2006; **102:** 16–17.
- Peace G. Integrated cancer care: linking medicine and therapies. *Nurs Times*. 2002; **98:** 35–7.
- Werneke U. A guide to using complementary alternative medicines in cancer. *Nurs Times*. 2005; **101:** 32–5.

Part 3

The problem of pain

Some definitions of words associated with pain

There are a number of words associated with pain in its many types and presentations, and it is necessary to know what they mean. There are several definitions of pain, but this is the one we prefer, because it reminds us that pain is not just a physical sensation.

> Pain is an unpleasant sensory and emotional experience associated with actual or potential tissue damage, or it is described in terms of such damage.
>
> (International Association for the Study of Pain, 1994)[1]

Other definitions associated with pain are now offered in alphabetical order.

Allodynia is pain caused by a stimulus that does not normally result in pain.
Analgesia is the absence of pain during exposure to a stimulus that would normally result in pain.
Causalgia is a syndrome consisting of a mixture of sustained burning pain, allodynia and increased sensitivity to stimuli as a result of nerve damage.
Central pain is pain associated with damage to the brain and spinal cord.
Dysaesthesia is an unpleasant sensation which can result from a stimulus or which may arise spontaneously.
Hyperaesthesia is increased sensitivity to a sensation.
Hyperalgesia in an increased response to a painful stimulus.
Hyperpathia is an exaggerated subjective response to painful stimuli, with a continuing sensation of pain after the stimulation has ceased.
Neuralgia is pain in the distribution of a nerve.
Neuropathy is a disturbance of normal nerve function.
Neuropathic pain is pain transmitted by a damaged nerve pathway. It is usually only partly opioid sensitive.
Nociceptors are receptors that respond to unpleasant stimuli.
Nociceptive pain is pain transmitted by an intact nerve. It is usually opioid sensitive.
Pain threshold is the least amount of pain recognised.
Pain tolerance level is the greatest amount of pain that can be tolerated.

Reference

1 Merskey H and Bogduk N eds. *Classification of Chronic Pain, Second Edition.* Seattle: IASP Press; 1994.

Chapter 13

Pain assessment

> All pain is one malady with many names.
>
> Antiphanes (*c*.408–*c*.334 BC), Greek philosopher

Introduction

Pain is more than just the physical component, and needs to be assessed with regard to all of its aspects and presentations.

The concept of 'total pain' reminds us of the various components of pain:

- physical – the element of pain that responds to analgesia
- psychological – the 'hurting' that one experiences as a result of illness
- social – loss of job, social position, role in family, work, etc.
- spiritual – what is the meaning of it all, why is God doing this to me? etc.

Pain may be due to many causes other than malignancy. Arthritis still causes pain, even when cancer is present, but it is easy to overlook other causes of pain and focus on the cancer as the sole cause.

Other things to remember when assessing pain include the following:

- each type of pain has its own specific characteristics
- multiple pains may be present at the same time
- the amount of pain experienced varies both from person to person and according to the circumstances
- tolerance of pain varies from person to person.

C Consider

When assessing pain, think about the patient's pain in terms of the following:

- cause or causes (e.g. related to cancer, treatment or non-malignant disease)
- intensity, site, nature, distribution and duration of each pain that they have
- past experience of pain
- understanding – what does the pain mean to the patient?

Pain in cancer can be caused by:

- cancer – either the primary tumour or secondary spread
- concurrent non-malignant disorder.

The pain may be related to:

- cancer or debility (e.g. muscle spasm, constipation or pressure areas)
- treatment (e.g. chemotherapy-induced peripheral neuropathy).

Many patients with advanced cancer have multiple pains from several of these categories, each of which can be influenced by mood and morale.

A Assess

The letters PQRST originally used by Twycross can be used to remind us that when assessing pain we should consider the following aspects. We have added U and V.

P	**P**alliating and **P**rovoking agents
Q	**Q**uality of the pain
R	**R**adiation – where it is and where it goes
S	**S**everity
T	**T**iming – intermittent or constant
U	**U**nique to the individual, not specific to their diagnosis or disease status
V	**V**ariable, depending on many factors (e.g. mood, morale, etc.).

- Ask the patient to describe the pain. If the patient is unable to do this, invite the opinions of the family and members of the multi-professional team to tell you how the patient has been behaving, which might indicate the pain site and severity. Repeat this for each pain.
- Assess the patient's behaviour, looking for non-verbal cues.
- Examine the patient, paying specific attention to the local pain site(s) and looking for a more general disease process as the cause of pain.
- Investigate each pain appropriately (e.g. with X-rays if a bony secondary is suspected).
- Review current management regularly, preferably at least every 24 hours.

℞ Remedy

Published reports indicate that about 70% of cancer patients are experiencing pain or being treated for it. Accurate diagnosis of the cause of the pain is essential before one can select the appropriate analgesic. This is discussed in the following chapters.

E Extra information

Most patients who have pain associated with advanced cancer experience multiple pains. Several studies have demonstrated an average of three different pains in many patients, and four in a significant percentage.

Accurate recording of the patient's pain(s) and of the response to interventions is important. To facilitate this, the use of body diagrams (*see* Figure 13.1) and a pain assessment tool can be invaluable.

The position of each pain should be recorded, and the severity of each should be documented. Use different colours to allow easy identification.

Other available tools that can be used by children or patients with a communication difficulty include the *Wong and Baker Faces Rating Scale* (*see* Figure 13.2)[1] and the *Faces Pain Scale* (*see* Figure 13.3).[2]

Although these two scales were developed for use in children, they can be used in adults who have difficulty in communication or learning disability.

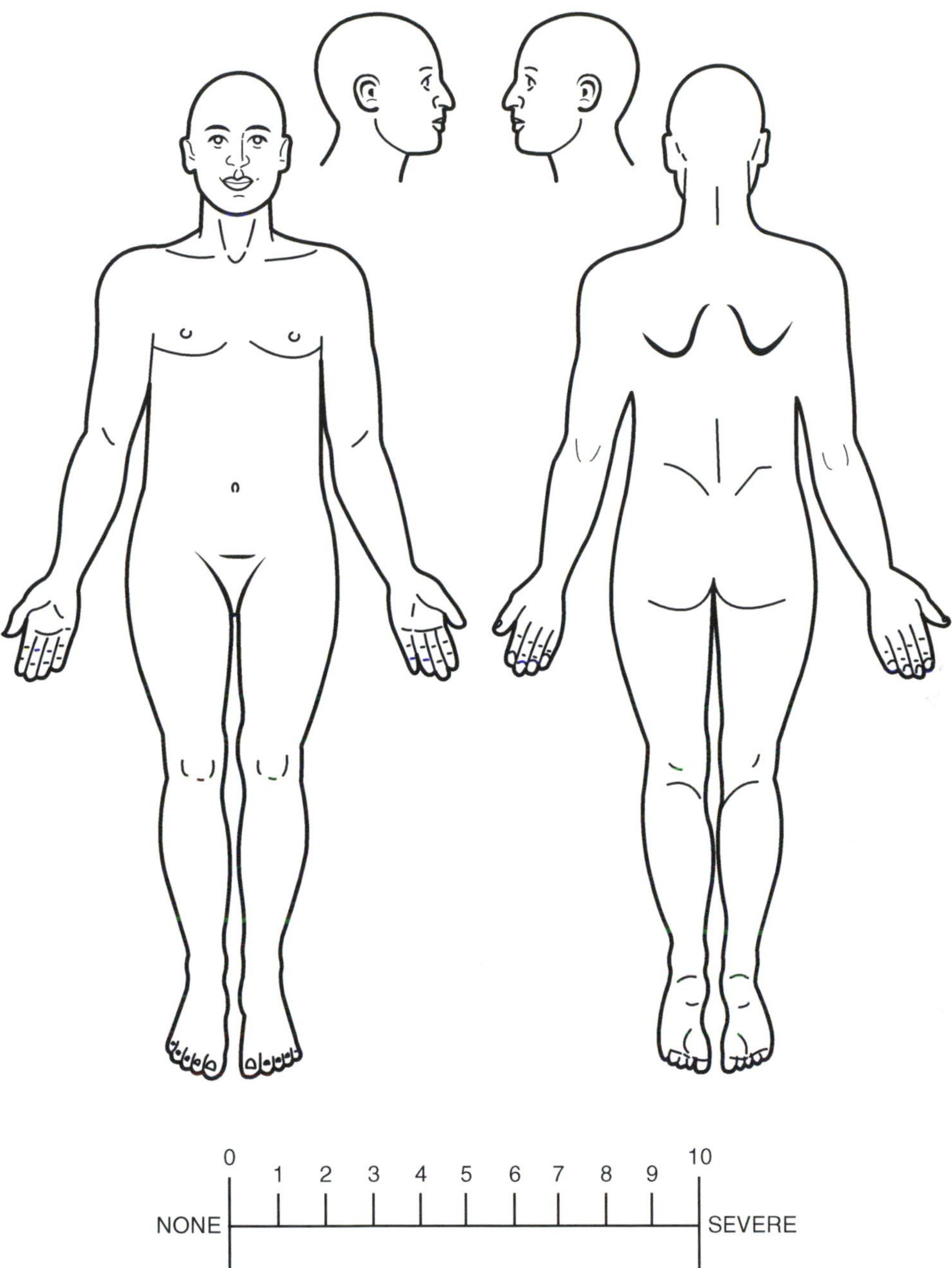

Figure 13.1 Body diagram for recording site and severity of pain.

Several words may be used to describe the pain. Here are some that were recorded by a selection of patients. They illustrate how variable the experience of pain can be.

> Aching, annoying, blinding, burning, cutting, dull, gnawing, hurting, intense, miserable, piercing, sickening, stinging, tender, throbbing, torture, unbearable, vicious.

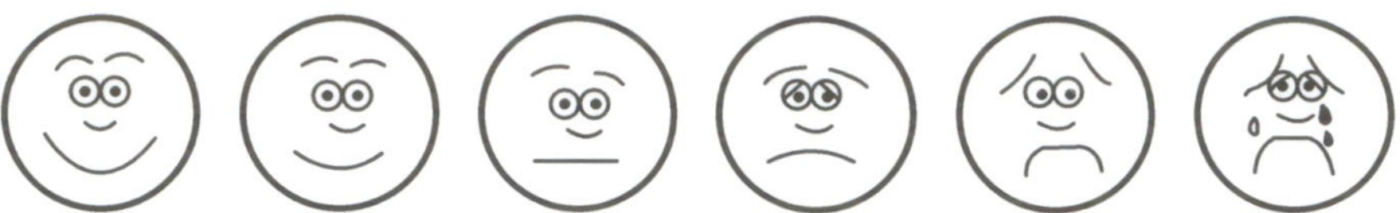

Figure 13.2 Wong and Baker Faces Rating Scale.[1]

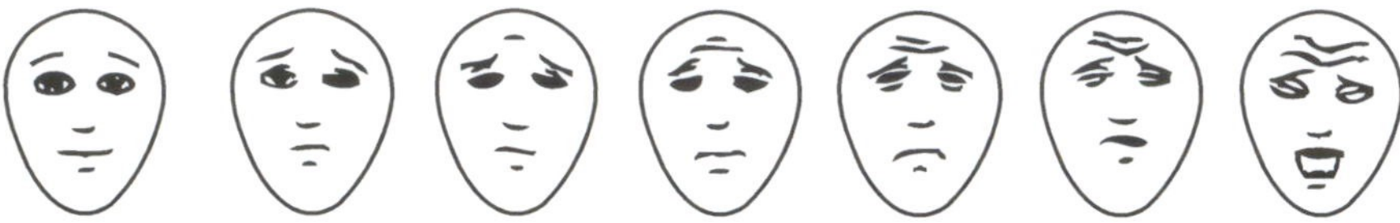

Figure 13.3 Faces Pain Scale.[2]

In addition to the physical pain, it is important to remember that a sense of hopelessness and a fear of impending death may be present, adding to the total suffering of the cancer patient.

References

1 Wong D, Baker C. Pain in children: comparison of assessment scales. *Paediatr Nurse.* 1988; **14:** 9–17.
2 Bieri D *et al.* The Faces Pain Scale for the self-assessment of the severity of pain experienced by children: development, initial validation and preliminary investigation for ratio scale properties. *Pain.* 1990; **41:** 139–50.

Further reading

This book deals primarily with the management of pain in adults. Paediatric pain management and pain management in the elderly are discussed in the following references.

- Twycross A, Moriarty A, Betts T. *Paediatric Pain Management: a multi-disciplinary approach.* Oxford: Radcliffe Medical Press; 1998.
- Morrison RS, Meier DE, editors. *Geriatric Palliative Care.* Oxford: Oxford University Press; 2003.

Chapter 14

Treatment options for managing pain

> The silliest charm gives more comfort to thousands in sorrow and pain than they will ever get from the knowledge that proves it foolish and vain.
>
> Irish proverb

Introduction

There may be more than one cause of the pain, and some pains may be due to conditions other than the cancer. Cancer pains may therefore be divided into opioid-responsive pain and opioid-non-responsive pain.

There are several factors that affect pain perception, and pain is very variable, so assessment and review need to be carried out regularly, with the drug given and the dose titrated to the response.

C Consider

- Who is the best person to monitor the patient's pain? Can the patient do this reliably by him- or herself?
- What is the response to previous or current analgesia?
- What is the range of treatment modalities available locally?
- What is the patient's attitude towards being offered the different treatment modalities available?

What is the patient's emotional and spiritual state? This alters their perception of pain and their ability to cope.

A Assess

If a pain assessment has not been carried out, it must be done now.

℞ Remedy

Having made an adequate assessment, you should then prescribe according to the type and severity of pain using the six basic principles advised by the World Health Organization (WHO) when prescribing for opioid-responsive pains.

1. Give drugs by mouth whenever feasible.
2. Give drugs by the clock (i.e. regularly).
3. Give drugs by the analgesic ladder.
4. Prescribe for the individual.
5. Use adjuvants as appropriate.
6. Give drugs with attention to detail.

Give drugs by mouth whenever feasible

Oral morphine is the strong opioid of choice for cancer pain. It has a variable plasma half-life, usually between 1½ and 2½ hours, and provides effective analgesia for up to 4 hours. With the exception of patients with renal failure, there is no danger of drug accumulation. In practice, the choice of prescribing lies between aqueous solution of morphine sulphate/hydrochloride (4-hourly), immediate-release tablets (4-hourly) and modified-release tablets or suspension.

Modified-release preparations are available with a 12-hour or 24-hour duration of action. It is essential that the patient is made aware that the tablets must be taken at 12- or 24-hour intervals in order to avoid accumulation or washout from irregular or badly timed doses.

Give drugs by the clock

Analgesics should be given on a regular basis. The next dose should be given before the effect of the previous one has completely worn off. To do this effectively, one must know the duration of action of the preparation that is being prescribed.

Give drugs by the analgesic ladder

The WHO has established an analgesic ladder (steps 1 to 3 below) based on the premise that if a drug ceases to be effective, it is pointless to give an alternative drug of similar strength, but rather one should prescribe a drug that is definitely stronger. To achieve this, one progresses from step 1 to step 3 of the analgesic ladder appropriate to the needs of the patient for effective pain management. The WHO analgesic ladder has been modified to a 5-step plan, taking account of newer modalities.

5 Intrathecal or epidural opioids ± step 3 drugs

4 Spinal opioids ± step 3 drugs

3 Strong opioid ± non-opioid ± adjuvants

2 Weak opioid ± non-opioid ± adjuvants

1 Non-opioid ± adjuvants

Initial cancer pain →→→ Increasing cancer pain →→→ Refractory cancer pain

Figure 14.1 The WHO analgesic ladder.

Prescribe for the individual

There is no 'standard dose' of morphine that can be universally applied when treating cancer pain. The correct dose for the individual patient is that which relieves their pain without causing unacceptable side-effects.

Perhaps the pain is due to fear of increasing the opioid dose or fear of addiction expressed by both patient and professional. Both fears are unfounded. The rule is to tailor the opioid dose to the needs of the individual.

The dose of morphine required by each cancer patient will vary and must therefore be individualised. Whereas non-opioid drugs and the weak opioids have a 'ceiling' above which an increase in dose does not confer any extra analgesia, this is not true of the strong opioids, such as morphine, which have no maximum dose. The dose ultimately required must be attained by titration of the dose against the intensity of the individual's pain.

The simplest method of dose administration is to use 4-hourly morphine in an instant-release formulation, and the same dose for breakthrough pain. This breakthrough dose may be given as frequently as required, and the total daily dose of morphine can be reviewed at daily intervals. The regular 4-hourly dose may then be adjusted according to how many breakthrough doses have been given.

The average patient may require a starting dose of 10 mg of morphine mixture 4-hourly or 30 mg of modified-release morphine 12-hourly.

Starting doses are generally lower in the elderly, in children and in the presence of severe liver disease. Similarly, people with impaired renal function are more sensitive to morphine and are more likely to develop toxic side-effects.

To decide the correct dose when prescribing a strong opioid for the first time, the potency of the current medication should be compared with morphine which is the standard.

Some common weak opioids are listed here and their potency compared with that of morphine. These comparisons only apply to morphine in doses of up to about 10 mg, and are only intended as a guide.

Analgesic	**Potency compared with morphine**
Codeine	1/10
Dihydrocodeine	1/8

A simple example will illustrate the principle of effective prescribing. Assume that a patient is taking a combined preparation containing acetaminophen (paracetamol) 500 mg and codeine 30 mg per tablet. If the patient is taking the maximum recommended dose of eight tablets per 24 hours, this compares as follows.

$$8 \times 30 \text{ mg codeine} = 240 \text{ mg codeine per 24 hours}$$

The potency of codeine is 1/10 of that of morphine. Therefore the equivalent dose of morphine per 24 hours required to achieve the same analgesia is 24 mg. This should be considered when prescribing, and a realistic prescription would be to give modified-release morphine at a dose of 15 mg 12-hourly. This exercise should be done before starting patients on morphine in order to determine a realistic starting dose.

Co-proxamol, a combination of dextropropoxyphene and acetaminophen (paracetamol), is currently being withdrawn in the UK. Some manufacturers have already withdrawn the drug, and it is anticipated that withdrawal will be complete by the end of 2007.[1]

Use adjuvants as appropriate

Adjuvant analgesics are a diverse group of drugs, some of which have no conventional analgesic activity. Nevertheless, their actions may complement or supplant those of conventional analgesics. Some adjuvants may have a synergistic effect, and adjuvant analgesics should not be prescribed routinely. The choice of drug is always dictated by the needs of the individual patient.

Some examples of adjuvants include the following:

- *antibiotics* in pain due to infection
- *anticonvulsants* in lancinating (shooting, stabbing) nerve pain (due to nerve destruction rather than compression). The probable mode of action is the suppression of unwanted pain impulses produced in the damaged nerve tissue
- *antidepressants* in dysaesthetic (e.g. superficial burning) nerve pain. The mode of action is uncertain, but may be due to the blocking of synaptic neurotransmitter chemicals involved in central pain transmission
- *corticosteroids* (e.g. dexamethasone) in nerve compression, spinal cord compression, headaches due to raised intracranial pressure, and hepatomegaly. The probable mode of action is the action of the steroid in reducing peritumour oedema
- *muscle relaxants* in pain of skeletal muscle spasm
- *nerve blocks* and other neurological procedures can be effective when opioids fail
- *non-steroidal anti-inflammatory drugs (NSAIDs)* in bone pain. Gastric protection should be considered
- *palliative radiotherapy*. A short course of radiotherapy may have an important role in treating pain due to primary and secondary cancer. Such courses should not produce side-effects. The advice of a radiotherapist or clinical oncologist should be sought.

Pain due to bony secondary deposits responds to radiotherapy in up to 90% of cases. Complete control of pain is achieved in 50–60% of cases. Onset of pain relief may occur within 2–3 days, but maximum benefits are seen at 2–3 weeks. Often only one fraction of radiotherapy will be required. Because the effect is not immediate, adequate analgesia should be offered and regularly reviewed, and opioid doses reduced as pain resolves. In addition to bone pain, pain due to local recurrence (e.g. in rectal cancer or other pelvic tumours) and pain due to Pancoast's tumour of the lung may respond to palliative radiotherapy.

- *Palliative radiotherapy* may have other useful effects in the treatment of patients with advanced cancer. It can be used for the following:
  - fungating breast cancer
  - haematuria in advanced bladder cancer
  - haemoptysis in lung cancer.
- *TENS (transcutaneous electrical nerve stimulation)* may help.
- *Complementary therapies* may also have a role to play. These include:
  - acupuncture
  - distraction
  - hypnosis
  - imagery
  - reflexology
  - relaxation therapies.

Other complementary therapies may be requested by the patient. These can be helpful and should be considered for comfort if nothing else.

Give drugs with attention to detail

Explore the patient's total pain and deal with all of the aspects. One of the barriers to effective pain management is a lack of understanding – both of what is happening and sometimes of how to achieve effective pain relief. This can be minimised by effective communication.

E Extra information

Pain in advancing disease is likely to increase, so regular assessment and adjustment of the analgesic dose are essential. Such a need for increased analgesia due to advancing disease does not imply addiction.

One-third of advanced cancer patients do not experience pain. For the remaining two-thirds, pain relief can be achieved in about nine out of ten patients.

Transdermal delivery systems using skin patches (e.g. fentanyl) are available. These have a long half-life and should only be used when pain is controlled and the dose is stable. The patch is usually only changed every third day. This avoids the need for regular oral medication, although breakthrough medication, in the form of instant-release morphine, must be prescribed in the usual way.

Reference

1 Anon. Withdrawal of co-proxamol (Distalgesic, Cosalgesic, Dolgesic). *Curr Probl Pharmacovigilance.* 2006; **31:** 11.

Further reading

- Aitkenhead SM. The role of the nurse consultant in managing paediatric pain. *Prof Nurse.* 2003; **19:** 49–52.
- Barrie J. The value of thorough assessment in the management of cancer pain. *Prof Nurse.* 2004; **19:** 446–8.
- Blackburn D, Somerville E, Squire S. Methadone: an alternative conversion regime. *Eur J Palliat Care.* 2002; **9:** 93–6.
- Campbell W. Therapeutic options in the drug management of nociceptive pain. *Prescriber.* 2004; **15:** 54–64.
- Closs SJ. What can be done to meet the needs of older people experiencing pain? *Prof Nurse.* 2004; **20:** 29–31.
- Davis C. A new 24-hour hydrogel suppository. *Eur J Palliat Care.* 2000; **7:** 165–7.
- Fallon M, Hanks G, Cherny N. Principles of control of cancer pain. *BMJ.* 2006; **332:** 1022–4.
- Lefebvre-Chapiro S and the DOLOPLUS Group. The DOLOPLUS 2 scale – evaluating pain in the elderly. *Eur J Palliat Care.* 2001; **8:** 191–4.
- McLoughlin C. Opioids. *Prof Nurse.* 2004; **19:** 51–2.
- Needham J. Issues relating to effective pain management in young people. *Prof Nurse.* 2004; **19:** 406–8.
- Radbruch L. Efficacy and tolerability of buprenorphine TDS in cancer pain patients. *Eur J Palliat Care.* 2003; **10:** 13–16.
- Shah S, Hardy J. Oxycodone: a review of the literature. *Eur J Palliat Care.* 2001; **8:** 93–6.

- Shaw P. The use of NSAIDs in patients with cancer: just how safe is it? *Eur J Palliat Care.* 2001; **8:** 181–5.
- Strohscheer I. Oral ketamine in patients with difficult cancer pain. *Eur J Palliat Care.* 2005; **12:** 54–6.
- Valera J-P, Aubry R. Morphine – doctors' beliefs and the myths. *Eur J Palliat Care.* 2000; **7:** 178–82.
- Vielvoye-Kerkmeer A. Long-term treatment with buprenorphine TDS in patients with chronic pain. *Eur J Palliat Care.* 2003; **10:** 17–19.
- Vielvoye-Kerkmeer A *et al.* Sustained-release morphine sulphate in cancer pain. *Eur J Palliat Care.* 2002; **9:** 137–40.

Chapter 15

Pain that persists or becomes out of control

> The immediate origins of misery and suffering need immediate attention. The old methods of care and caring had to be rediscovered and the best of modern medicine had to be turned to the task of new study and therapy specifically directed at pain.
>
> Patrick Wall[1]

Introduction

Sometimes the patient continues to experience pain despite assessment and treatment. There are several possibilities. The pain may not have been fully assessed, either because a cue was missed or because the patient did not report having more than one type of pain. Some patients are anxious about the numbers of tablets they are taking and hope that one opioid will cure all types of pain, which is not the case. Either way, the first place to start is with reassessment.

C Consider

Is this a new pain, or a pain that was present before which was not reported or which was thought to be responsive to the analgesia prescribed?

Think about the pain assessment that was carried out and consider the following:

- was adequate assessment carried out?
- were all aspects of the patient's pain assessed?
- was appropriate and adequate treatment prescribed?
- were coexisting conditions that might affect pain perception considered?
- were concurrent non-malignant causes assessed?

Think about the possible causes of continuing pain or a new pain:

- debility
- disease progression
- treatment side-effects (e.g. constipation)
- more than one pain, previously not reported
- poor patient compliance due to fears about drug side-effects.

Think about the expectations of the patient, the family and professional carers.

- Are the patient's expectations about treatment being met?
- Are the patient's expectations about treatment realistic?
- Has the patient understood and followed the instructions about treatment?
- How does the relatives' perception of the patient's pain match your own perception?
- Is there any problem within the team with regard to pain assessment and management?

A Assess

Is the patient getting the drug at all, or in adequate doses? Assess the following:

- absorption. Is the drug not being absorbed due to vomiting, faulty adhesion of a transdermal patch or failure of subcutaneous infusion or other equipment?
- breakthrough pain requiring medication
- compliance. Fear of addiction to opioids in cancer pain relief is common but unfounded. Reassurance is essential.

Reassess the pain using the PQRSTUV principles described in Chapter 13 (*see* page 54).

Examine the patient, assessing their mood and morale and looking for signs of anxiety or depression as you talk to them. Look for the following:

- motor weakness
- neurological problems
- signs of enlarged organs causing pressure
- skin problems over pressure points, particularly in debilitated patients
- tenderness at sites of known metastases, particularly bone metastases.

Review the results of previous investigations that may help in the management of pain (e.g. X-rays, bone scans).

℞ Remedy

An accurate diagnosis is essential for the effective treatment of cancer pain. Making an accurate diagnosis requires an understanding of pathology, anatomy with regard to referred pain, and patterns of metastatic spread.

Breakthrough pain

'Breakthrough pain' is the term used to describe pain that occurs when patients are receiving regular analgesia for pain. There are some basic rules to observe when prescribing an opioid to manage breakthrough pain.

- The dose of opioid for a breakthrough pain is equivalent to approximately *one-sixth* of the total 24-hour dose.
- If the breakthrough dose is required frequently (more than twice in 24 hours), reassess the patient to diagnose the reason. It is usually due to progression of the disease.
- The breakthrough doses needed should be taken into account when the prescription of the main analgesic is reviewed. Calculate the new dose by adding the total given for breakthrough to the total 24-hour dose that is already being given, to calculate the new minimum opioid dose required per 24 hours (i.e. total dose per 24 hours plus breakthrough doses in previous 24 hours equals the minimum dose required to keep pain under control). In practice, it makes sense to round this up to the nearest convenient dose to prescribe, especially if you are using sustained-release preparations.
- Remember to increase the breakthrough dose when you increase the dose of the main analgesic.

- If the patient is on continuous subcutaneous infusion, the breakthrough dose of opioid should be given subcutaneously.
- Don't forget to review the laxative dose when opioid doses are increased.

Some common causes of pain and their management

- *Opioid-responsive* pains include visceral pain.
- *Opioid-poorly-responsive* pains include:
  - bone pain (use an NSAID alone or in addition)
  - nerve compression – prescribe corticosteroid + opioid.
- *Opioid-resistant* pains include:
  - muscle spasm – prescribe a muscle relaxant
  - nerve damage pain – prescribe an anticonvulsant and/or antidepressant.

Opioid-responsive pain

- Give immediate pain relief (e.g. bolus subcutaneous injection of diamorphine) if the pain is opioid responsive.
- Review after a short period (e.g. 1 hour).
- Discuss the cause of the pain and the treatment plan with the patient, setting realistic and achievable goals of pain control.
- Prescribe appropriate treatment (including breakthrough pain medication) for 24 hours, and remind the patient of the need for the full doses to be taken at the regular prescribed intervals.
- Reassess the patient every 24 hours and make appropriate adjustments until they are pain-free.
- Keep the patient, the family and other professionals informed and updated about the changes, and make sure that any problems are reported promptly.

Opioid-poorly-responsive and opioid-resistant pain

- Consider the use of adjuvants, such as dexamethasone, in patients with headaches due to increased intracranial pressure.
- Consider the use of non-drug measures, such as radiotherapy, in patients with bone metastases.

If appropriate, consult with specific caring professionals, such as radiotherapists, anaesthetic service, pain clinics and physiotherapists, about palliative radiotherapy as nerve blocks (e.g. coeliac plexus block in painful pancreatic, gastric or biliary cancers). The opioid dose will probably need to be reduced quite substantially following such successful procedures. If such a procedure is to be undertaken, switch the patient from modified-release opioids to an instant-release preparation given every 4 hours, and be prepared to reduce the doses quite quickly in order to minimise the risk of overdosing.

Consider the use of complementary therapies or self-help strategies.

What if the patient cannot take morphine?

If pain is opioid-responsive, but for some reason the patient cannot take morphine, there are alternatives. These are discussed below.

Fentanyl

Morphine acts on the μ_1- and μ_2-receptors. Fentanyl acts more selectively on only the μ_1-receptor. It will relieve opioid-sensitive pain and may cause fewer side-effects such as constipation and dysphoria. Because it is not absorbed orally, it must be given by injection (which has a very short duration of action) or as a transdermal patch.

Indications for considering the use of fentanyl include the following:

- there is adequate analgesia but unacceptable side-effects with morphine
- the oral route is not suitable or acceptable, the pain is controlled and the opioid requirement is stable, in which case fentanyl patches are suitable
- renal impairment is leading to the accumulation of morphine metabolites.

Difficulties associated with the use of fentanyl include the following:

- dose conversion from morphine to fentanyl can be complicated. Check the dose very carefully
- toxicity due to fentanyl is less easy to spot than morphine toxicity because of the lack of hallucinations. Symptoms may be very subtle, including feeling generally unwell, or mild drowsiness.

Hydromorphone

Hydromorphone is very similar to morphine, but its metabolites may cause fewer side-effects in patients with renal impairment. Given orally it is approximately 7.5 times as potent as morphine.

Indications for considering the use of hydromorphone include the following:

- renal impairment
- unacceptable side-effects, notably confusion and hallucinations, but with good pain relief with morphine.

Oxycodone

Oxycodone is a strong opioid similar to morphine. Receptor-binding activity is not clearly defined. The dose required is 50% of that of morphine for the same analgesic action. It causes less vomiting but more constipation than morphine.

Indications for considering the use of oxycodone include the following:

- patients who are allergic to morphine.

Difficulties associated with the use of oxycodone include the following:

- some patients have a genetic inability to adequately metabolise the drug and may not obtain full analgesia.

Methadone

Methadone is an agonist at the μ- and δ-opioid receptors. It has a very long and variable half-life (8–60 hours) and may take up to 10 days to reach a steady state in the plasma. There is a tendency for the drug to accumulate in the elderly and those with liver failure.

Indications for considering the use of methadone include the following:

- morphine tolerance
- partial response to morphine (e.g. neuropathic pain).

Difficulties associated with the use of methadone include the following:

- the dose must be reassessed, and usually reduced, a few days after starting methadone
- careful and regular assessment is essential, as accumulation may occur up to 10 days afterwards.

E Extra information

Combined preparations

The question sometimes arises as to whether the combined drugs such as co-codamol offer any benefit over single agents such as paracetamol (acetaminophen). The answer is that combined preparations are beneficial if the two drugs have different modes of action, such as a weak opioid and a NSAID in combination.

Around 10% of the codeine in co-codamol is converted to morphine in the body and adds to the effect of the paracetamol.

In practice, it is better to titrate the individual drugs to the response, but this often means that the patient needs to take more tablets, and this may result in poor compliance.

Myths about opioids

All drugs have some side-effects, and opioids are no exception. There are many myths associated with morphine as well, so some of the issues that one may have to deal with are described below.

Clouding of consciousness

In the first few days of treatment while dosages are being established there may be some sedation. This settles quickly as doses are adjusted to individual needs. Similarly, nausea should not last longer than a few days during the initial stages of dose titration.

Dependence

Psychological dependence (addiction) does not usually occur in patients who are prescribed morphine for cancer pain, provided that it is used in the context of total patient care.

Physical dependence (the development of a withdrawal reaction on abrupt dosage reduction or stopping morphine) may be seen. This is an intrinsic property of opioids. Such an unpleasant situation can be avoided by not withdrawing opioids suddenly.

Sometimes a reduction in opioid doses is required (e.g. after a successful nerve block). In such cases, using an instant-release preparation with a short half-life allows doses to be safely reduced over a period of days. This avoids the risk of either sudden withdrawal or short-term overdosing.

Respiratory depression and hastening death

Clinically significant respiratory depression is not a feature of morphine prescribed for cancer pain, even in patients with established pulmonary disease. When prescribed at the correct doses, the morphine is fully utilised at the receptor sites.

In several studies, conducted over significant time periods, there was no evidence that morphine prescribed at the correct dose shortens life.

Tolerance

Some patients fear that if they start taking morphine early in their pain experience, there will be nothing strong enough available later. However, as there is no ceiling effect with morphine, this is not the case.

Reference

1 Wall P. Editorial. *Pain.* 1986; **25(1):** 1–4.

Further reading

- Barrie J. The role of the nurse in the management of breakthrough pain in cancer. *Eur J Palliat Care.* 2005; **12**(5): **(Suppl.):** 8–10.
- Campbell W, Broomhead C. Managing severe pain. *Prescriber.* 2006; **17:** 43–4.
- Colvin L, Forbes K, Fallon M. Difficult pain. *BMJ.* 2006; **332:** 1081–4.
- Davies A. Current thinking in cancer breakthrough pain management. *Eur J Palliat Care.* 2005; **12**(5): **(Suppl.):** 4–6.
- Davies A, editor. *Cancer-Related Breakthrough Pain.* Oxford: Oxford University Press; 2006.
- Fallon M, Hanks G, Cherny N. Principles of control of cancer pain. *BMJ.* 2006; **332:** 1022–4.
- Guindon C *et al.* Terminal cancer pain. *Eur J Palliat Care.* 2001; **8:** 49–53.
- Hanks G. Oral transmucosal fentanyl citrate for the management of breakthrough pain. *Eur J Palliat Care.* 2001; **8:** 6–9.
- Hanks G. Breakthrough pain in cancer. *Eur J Palliat Care.* 2005; **12**(5): **(Suppl.):** 3–4.
- Middleton C. Barriers to the provision of effective pain management. *Nurs Times.* 2004; **100:** 42–5.
- Nugent M. The management of breakthrough cancer pain: is current practice best practice? *Eur J Palliat Care.* 2006; **13:** 10–12.
- Shah S, Hardy J. Oxycodone: a review of the literature. *Eur J Palliat Care.* 2001; **8:** 93–6.
- Sherder E *et al.* Recent developments in pain in dementia. *BMJ.* 2005; **330:** 461–4.
- Strohscheer I. Oral ketamine in patients with difficult cancer pain. *Eur J Palliat Care.* 2005; **12:** 54–6.
- Vielvoye Kerkmeer A *et al.* Sustained-release morphine sulphate in cancer pain. *Eur J Palliat Care.* 2002; **9:** 137–40.
- Zeppetella J. Is the recommended titration schedule for OTFC (oral transmucosal fentanyl citrate) too conservative? *Eur J Palliat Care.* 2005; **12**(5): **(Suppl.):** 6–7.

Chapter 16

Bone pain

Where a man feels pain, he lays his hand.

Dutch proverb

Introduction

Breast tumours are by far the most common tumours that produce osteolytic lesions and weakness or fracture of the bones. Breast cancer accounts for nearly half of the fractures seen in cancer patients.

Bronchial carcinoma, prostate cancer and myeloma are also common causes, but almost any primary tumour can occasionally produce a pathological fracture.

C Consider

- Does the patient have one of the cancers commonly associated with bone secondaries?
- Has the disease progressed to involve bone? Bone metastases are a common cause of cancer pain.
- Did the pain start suddenly?
- How much does the pain affect activities of daily living?
- What does the patient think is going on?

A Assess

- Is there a pathological fracture?
- Is there any local tenderness over the affected bone? Bone lesions tend to produce well-localised pain. Patients will often point with one finger to the spot where they have pain. With muscle pain they often rub the affected area, and with nerve pain they often will not touch the area at all.
- Is there any involvement of the spine, evidenced by back or rib pain, or signs of cord compression (e.g. weakness of the leg, leg pain, paraesthesia, or urinary disturbance)?

Confirm the diagnosis with:

- a plain X-ray of the whole bone involved
- an MRI scan if possible, or
- a radioisotope scan of the whole skeleton, which will also define any further occult lesions.

℞ Remedy

Key elements in bone pain management are as follows:

- drug treatment, non-steroidal anti-inflammatory drugs (NSAIDs) and opioids
- radiotherapy – the treatment of choice
- surgery in selected cases.

It is important to realise that bone pain is poorly responsive to morphine. In metastatic bone disease the tumour cells often produce a high local concentration of prostaglandins. NSAIDs provide pain relief by blocking prostaglandin biosynthesis, which is part of the inflammatory response. Prostaglandins also heighten the sensation of pain. NSAIDs have anti-inflammatory, analgesic and antipyretic effects.

There is variability in the effectiveness of NSAIDs. If one NSAID does not help, it is worth trying another. There is no known reason for this phenomenon.

NSAIDs should be used with caution in renal impairment, and discontinued if there is evidence of deteriorating renal function.

Immediate control of pain

Use an NSAID – for example, naproxen sodium 500 mg twice daily, flurbiprofen 100 mg twice daily, diclofenac sodium modified-release 75 mg 12-hourly or, if bone pain is very severe, consider using a parenteral NSAID (e.g. ketorolac), which may be given subcutaneously via a syringe driver.

If a particular NSAID is only poorly successful in controlling the pain, consider changing to another – it may work better. Think about the need for gastric protection.

Consider whether you have prescribed NSAIDs soon enough and in adequate doses to achieve pain control, pending the effect of palliative radiotherapy.

Morphine doses should be titrated against pain, and may need to be increased or decreased. Remember that laxatives will need to be increased if the opioid doses are increased.

Long-term control of pain

Palliative radiotherapy is the treatment of choice.

- Has the area been irradiated before?
- Has the patient's tumour responded to radiotherapy before?
- Obtain the opinion of the radiotherapist without delay.
- Consider the role of orthopaedic surgery, which is probably underused.

Hormonal treatment may be required (e.g. for prostatic and breast carcinomas). Seek advice from the oncologist.

Suspected spinal cord compression

Metastatic disease of the spine produces two major problems. First, pain may be severe, due to expansion of tumour within the vertebrae, which may also fracture and collapse. Secondly, erosion of a vertebral body can cause mechanical instability of the spine at one or more levels. Neurological deficit, due to compression of the spinal cord, cauda equina or nerve roots, could result from either expanding extradural deposits or spinal instability.

Where there is impending spinal cord compression, prescribe dexamethasone, 16 mg daily in divided doses, pending urgent consultation with a radiotherapist, orthopaedic surgeon or neurosurgeon. *These consultations are a matter of urgency* and should be arranged immediately. Unacceptable delay in referral results in preventable long-term immobility.

The patient and their family should be sensitively made aware that treatment is directed at relief of pain, restoration of mobility and return to independence with the minimum of delay.

When prescribing steroids, give the last dose in the early evening in order to avoid insomnia.

Orthopaedic treatment

Contact the orthopaedic surgeon without delay if there is a risk of pathological fracture of a long bone, or if there is vertebral involvement. The orthopaedic surgeon can offer a variety of options that might prevent a fracture and stabilise weak bones; their role is probably not fully appreciated and the service is probably used less than it should be due to failure to appreciate what can be offered.

Both the patient and their family need to be made aware that surgery for metastatic bone disease is not expected to prolong life or be in any way curative. It is a palliative procedure intended to control symptoms.

An orthopaedic surgeon may have various roles, including the following:

- decompression of the spinal cord
- fixation of pathological fracture
- stabilisation of the vertebral column.

When bone pain is present due to bone metastases, the possibility of hypercalcaemia must always be considered. The symptoms and signs of hypercalcaemia include the following:

- bone pain that is difficult to control
- confusion or drowsiness
- dehydration
- nausea and vomiting.

Bisphosphonates inhibit bone resorption, correct hypercalcaemia, reduce pain and prevent development of new osteolytic lesions. The incidence of fractures is reduced and quality of life is improved. Several of these drugs are licensed for this indication. Prophylactic use of bisphosphonates may be worth considering in patients at high risk from bone disease.

E Extra information

The role of palliative radiotherapy

As well as giving rapid pain control, the structural integrity of the bone may improve in the medium term, with recalcification at the site of the metastases.

External beam radiotherapy is the best treatment for *localised* metastatic bone pain. A single dose seems to be as effective as fractionated treatment, and is clearly more convenient.

Remember that radiotherapy may increase skin friability over the area that is being treated, and thus skin is more at risk from breakdown.

Reassess pain approximately 1 week after irradiation. Relief may not be experienced for 2 weeks, and other pain control must be offered until radiotherapy takes full effect.

Further reading

- Al-Hakim WI. The palliative role of orthopaedics. *BMJ.* 2006; **332:** 1227–8.
- Dewar JA. Managing metastatic bone pain. *BMJ.* 2004; **329:** 812–13.

Chapter 17

Nerve pain

> Illness is the doctor to whom we pay most heed; to kindness, to knowledge, we make promise only, pain we obey.
>
> M Proust (1871–1922)[1]

Introduction

Up to 40% of cancer patients experience neuropathic pain, which is pain that is transmitted by a damaged nerve system and is only partially responsive to opioids. It is difficult to treat, and more than one drug may be required to bring it under control.

Pain that appears to be neuropathic in origin may have a nociceptive opioid-responsive element as well.

C Consider

Nerve pain can result from four types of nerve involvement:

- compression of nerve tissue by tumour
- infiltration of nerve tissue by tumour
- treatment-related nerve damage
- unrelated illnesses causing nerve damage.

Compression and infiltration of nerve tissue may lead to:

- local nerve damage
- spinal cord or spinal nerve compression by the tumour.

Treatment-related nerve damage can be caused by:

- chemotherapy
- radiotherapy
- surgery.

Unrelated illnesses that may cause nerve damage include:

- diabetic neuropathy
- post-herpetic neuralgia.

A Assess

Assess the pain as outlined in the chapter on pain assessment. Decide the most likely cause of the pain.

Ask about the following:

- pain characteristics (e.g. allodynia, altered sensations, burning, hyperalgesia, neurological deficits, paraesthesia and tingling)
- sleep disruption due to the pain.

℞ Remedy

Neuropathic pain can be difficult to manage, and in order to ensure best compliance, it is always good practice to talk to the patient about the nature of neuropathic pain and to explain how it responds poorly to conventional painkillers, and that it may be necessary to try different therapies before an effective treatment is found. A paper published in the *New England Journal of Medicine* shows that combinations of drugs often work best.[2] Sadly, increasing the number of medications may result in poorer compliance.

There are a number of agents that may be tried for neuropathic pain. These include the following:

- acupuncture
- anticonvulsants
- capsaicin
- clonidine
- gabapentin
- ketamine
- methadone
- neurolytic procedures, cordotomy and nerve blocks
- NSAIDs
- opioids
- radiotherapy
- spinal injections – epidural and intrathecal
- steroids
- TENS
- tricyclic antidepressants.

Acupuncture

Acupuncture may be tried, with increased stimulation, or with the use of ultrasound or small electric currents. Evidence for how it works is not available, and the procedure must be used with care if there is a risk of bleeding or infection. Acupuncture should not be used on a limb affected by lymphoedema.

Anticonvulsants

Anticonvulsants act in a variety of ways and are traditionally used for lancinating and intermittent pain, but the evidence from published studies does not support this idea. There appears to be little to choose between antidepressants and anticonvulsants. All of the anticonvulsants should be used at their normal 'anticonvulsant' doses. They may take 6 weeks to become fully effective.

- Carbamazepine is widely used. It has several interactions, can be poorly tolerated by elderly patients, and should be slowly increased to the optimum dose to avoid side-effects.
- Clonazepam has been used and can be given subcutaneously.
- Gabapentin is the only drug licensed for all types of neuropathic pain. It appears to be well tolerated.
- Sodium valproate has been widely used, but reports on its effectiveness vary.

Capsaicin

Capsaicin is the chemical that causes the burning sensation associated with chillies. Tolerance of the taste develops as the capsaicin acts on the neurotransmitter substance P, inhibiting transmission of some pain impulses. It is used topically as a cream. It can sting, so should be applied carefully, wearing gloves. Broken skin and sensitive areas, including mucosal surfaces, should be avoided.

Clonidine

Clonidine, an α_2-adrenoreceptor agonist used to treat hypertension, has been shown to be effective in relieving neuropathic pain by acting at the level of the spinal cord. It acts synergistically with opioids, but its use may be limited by sedation and hypotension.

Gabapentin

Gabapentin works by blocking calcium channels, especially the $\alpha_2\delta$ channel. It is effective for a variety of nerve pain problems.

Gabapentin is sometimes combined with a tricyclic antidepressant when gabapentin alone is insufficient. The rationale for this is that they have different mechanisms of action.

Ketamine

Ketamine, a powerful analgesic anaesthetic, may be useful for neuropathic pain when used at sub-anaesthetic doses. Higher doses may also be useful for uncontrolled pain in the terminal stages. Ketamine can cause hallucinations, and expert advice should be sought before using this preparation.

Methadone

Methadone may be tried as a first-line opioid, but is more commonly used later when other opioids have failed.

Neurolytic procedures, cordotomy and nerve blocks

Cordotomy destroys the pain fibres in the spinal cord, and is used only for unilateral pain that is resistant to all other measures. The result is numbness and possible weakness, so this is not a procedure to be undertaken lightly.

Nerve blocks should be administered by an anaesthetist specialising in pain clinic work. A local anaesthetic is used first to ascertain the effect on the pain, and then a permanent blocking agent is used.

NSAIDs

NSAIDs are sometimes effective, probably by reducing associated inflammation or because the pain is of mixed aetiology. Patient responses and tolerance vary widely, and it may be necessary to try different NSAIDs in order to achieve maximum benefit.

Opioids

Opioids are sometimes used in cancer-related neuropathic pain because the pain may be of mixed aetiology with a nociceptive element, and because about one-third of neuropathic pains are opioid sensitive.

Fentanyl, tramodol and oxycodone may be more effective than morphine.

Radiotherapy

Radiotherapy can be used to reduce the bulk of tumour causing nerve compression. Pain may respond well, but some loss of function may remain.

Spinal injections: epidural and intrathecal

Epidural and intrathecal injections are administered by pain clinic anaesthetists. Direct delivery of opioids to the spinal cord is effective, reliable and reversible. Intrathecal opioids bind to the μ- and κ-receptors in the substantia gelatinosa of the spinal cord, but epidural opioids, which are not delivered as deeply, do so to a lesser extent.

Steroids

Dexamethasone is traditionally used. The mode of action is probably to reduce nerve sensitivity caused by inflammation, or to reduce peri-neural oedema. Start with a reasonably high dose of 8 mg daily, and then reduce the dose according to the response. Steroids should be used for as short a time as possible, and are helpful while other therapies such as radiotherapy or antidepressants are building up to their maximum effect.

TENS

TENS may be helpful for nerve pain. The only way to find out is by therapeutic trial. Certain pains, including post-herpetic neuralgia and pain in the head and neck area, are particularly amenable.

Avoid TENS if the patient has a cardiac pacemaker, and do not place electrodes on areas of vulnerable skin.

Tricyclic antidepressants

Tricyclic antidepressants act in several ways, including facilitation of the descending inhibitory pain pathways mediated by $5HT_3$ and noradrenaline. Amitriptyline (25–100 mg daily) or dosulepin (25–100 mg daily) may be helpful. Start with a lower dose of amitriptyline in the elderly. The doses required are generally less than those required for depression. Any tendency to cause drowsiness may be an added benefit. Lofepramine may be useful in frail elderly patients, starting with 70 mg at night.

Before starting on any of these drugs, patients should be made aware of certain essential facts.

- Neuropathic pain can be difficult to treat.
- Side-effects such as a dry mouth (e.g. with amitriptyline) are common.

- Some drugs take days or weeks to become fully effective.
- Unhelpful medications need to be phased out and stopped.
- Use of an antidepressant or anticonvulsant does not imply that the patient is depressed or that they are going to develop fits, and patients should be reassured about this.

Continue to reassess the patient regularly, paying attention to the following:

- satisfactory symptom control
- side-effects
- sleep.

E Extra information

'Deafferentation' is a particularly confusing term, which means different things to different people. It is an umbrella term encompassing a variety of quite different clinical syndromes. 'Nerve damage pain' or 'neuropathic pain' are preferable terms and are much more easily understood.

Nerve pain may present as superficial burning or as stabbing, shooting and excruciating pain. It may also present as a deep aching pain if there is an element of nerve compression.

No large randomised clinical trials have been conducted to assess the value of cannabis in neuropathic pain. However, two studies do suggest that cannabinoids reduce spasticity and neuropathic pain.[3]

References

1 Proust M. My social life. In: *Cities of the Plain.* London: Chatto and Windus. 1936.
2 Gilron I, Bailey JM, Dongsheng T *et al.* Morphine, gabapentin, or their combination for neuropathic pain. *New Engl J Med* 2005: **352:** 1324–34.
3 Wood S. Evidence for using cannabis and cannabinoids to manage pain. *Nurs Times.* 2004; **100:** 38–40.

Further reading

- Bennett M, editor. *Neuropathic Pain.* Oxford: Oxford University Press; 2006.
- Campbell W. First- and second-line treatments in neuropathic pain. *Prescriber.* 2005; **16:** 23–8.
- Hutchinson S. Neuropathic pain – the future is hopeful. *Forum.* 2005; **May issue:** 49–50.
- Johnson ME. Neuropathic pain in primary care. *New Generalist.* 2006; **4:** 27–30.
- Mishra S, Bhatnagar S. Managing phantom limb pain. *Eur J Palliat Care.* 2006; **13:** 54–6.
- Rocafort J, Viguria J. Gabapentin as an analgesic. *Eur J Palliat Care.* 2001; **8:** 54–6.

Chapter 18

The syringe driver

> Nature has placed mankind under the governance of two masters, pain and pleasure.
>
> Jeremy Bentham (1748–1832), English philosopher, *Introduction to the Principles of Morals and Legislation*

Introduction

While the oral route is to be preferred, there are times when it is not feasible or practical to use this route of administration for medications. Continuous subcutaneous infusion (CSCI) is very convenient, unobtrusive and acceptable.

Some patients may associate the use of CSCI with approaching death and nothing else. This myth should be dispelled.

Two syringe drivers are in common use. They are the Graseby® MS16A and the Graseby® MS26. A few key points are relevant here.

- Both deliver by length of the syringe barrel, not by volume.
- The MS16A delivers at a rate set in millimetres per hour.
- The MS26 delivers at a rate set in millimetres per 24 hours.

This makes the MS26 simpler and probably safer to set up and use. From now on, this text relates to the Graseby® MS26 syringe driver.

There is a 'boost button', but it is recommended that patients do not use this, for the following reasons:

- if there are other drugs as well as analgesics in the syringe, extra doses of these are being given as well, whether they are needed or not
- pressing the boost button and receiving bolus doses may cause local inflammation and pain
- the dose delivered per boost is inadequate as a breakthrough pain dose
- there is no lock-out period. The syringe driver delivers eight boosts and then alarms. Pressing the boost button again repeats this process
- unsupervised use of the boost button will result in premature delivery of the drug, which is of particular concern in a home setting, where one might only be checking the syringe driver once every 24 hours when refilling.

The syringe driver delivers by length, not volume. The MS26 can accommodate a syringe of 35 ml capacity and with a maximum travel distance of 60 mm. This is approximately 25 ml capacity. This becomes relevant if larger doses of prepared drugs are required.

A simple card can be designed to record relevant information, such as how different syringes vary in volume with regard to barrel length according to the manufacturer, and how long the first infusion will run, allowing for the volume used for priming the line when it is first set up.[1] This is particularly useful if different people will be responsible for setting up and refilling the syringe.

A simple chart can also be devised showing the drugs in the syringe, the time of set-up, and providing space in which to record remaining volume and the state of the skin at the infusion site, etc. This is useful for checking that the instrument is running properly.

C Consider

What are the indications for using a syringe driver?

First, the following are *not* indications:

- intractable pain
- nearing the end of life.

The main indications are easily divided into three groups, where the alternative routes of administration are either unavailable or unsuitable.

Intramuscular and intravenous

- Cachexia resulting in reduced muscle bulk when repeated IM injections are required.
- Discomfort and inconvenience of IV access.

Oral

- Dysphagia.
- Nausea and vomiting.
- Poor absorption by the oral route.
- Preferred route to reduce the number of oral medications required.
- Profound weakness and difficulty in swallowing.
- Unconsciousness.

Rectal

- Diarrhoea.
- Obstruction.
- Patient preference.

A Assess

In order to assess the need for and suitability of a syringe driver, examine the patient, paying attention to the following:

- physical symptoms
- psychological state, including fears about the use of a syringe driver.

Consider whether a syringe driver would overcome the difficulties associated with the following:

- ability to swallow
- compliance with medications
- confusion
- intestinal obstruction

- nausea and vomiting
- persisting fits
- profound weakness
- unacceptable numbers of tablets or large volumes of liquid medicines required.

℞ Remedy

What drugs can be used in a syringe driver and what are they used for?

The following drugs can all be used in a syringe driver.

Alfentanil

Alfentanil is a synthetic opioid, chemically related to fentanyl, and with strong agonist activity at the μ- and κ-receptors. It is suitable as an alternative to diamorphine in patients with renal failure. It is metabolised in the liver, so coexisting liver disease may necessitate a dose reduction. There is a possible interaction with erythromycin and ketoconazole, with resultant increased plasma levels of alfentanil.

Clonazepam

Clonazepam is a benzodiazepine derivative that is useful for anxiety, hiccup, myoclonic jerking, neuropathic pain, seizures and terminal agitation. Its administration by CSCI is supported by widespread use, but no trials supporting its use in a syringe driver were found. Phenobarbital and carbamazepine may interact, reducing the efficacy of clonazepam.

Cyclizine

Cyclizine is an antihistamine with antimuscarinic activity that is useful for nausea and vomiting. There is a theoretical risk of precipitation with several other drugs, and this can limit its use.

Dexamethasone

Dexamethasone is a steroid with a long half-life, so it is preferable to give it early in the day, by bolus dose, rather than by CSCI, in order to avoid sleep disruption. It is useful for breathlessness, headache or nausea and vomiting due to raised intracranial pressure, and for nerve compression pain. It may not mix with glycopyrronium, haloperidol and levomepromazine, with which it may form a precipitate. It interacts with anticonvulsants, resulting in a reduced serum level of dexamethasone.

Diamorphine

Diamorphine is the opioid of choice because it is about 13 times more soluble than morphine, allowing high doses to be given in very small volumes of fluid. It is stable with various other drugs when mixed in a syringe driver. It is about three times more potent than oral morphine. The metabolic breakdown products are excreted by the kidneys, so patients in renal failure are at greater risk of toxicity from morphine and diamorphine.

Diclofenac

Diclofenac is one of two NSAIDs that can be given by CSCI. It must not be used if there is a history of peptic ulceration or hypersensitivity to NSAIDs. It is useful for bone pain and biliary or renal colic. It can irritate the skin and must be given via a separate syringe driver.

Dihydrocodeine

Dihydrocodeine can be used in a syringe driver, but in practice this is rarely done. It appears to be stable in solution with midazolam and haloperidol. An exact conversion ratio has not been established, but the consensus appears to be that 60 mg of oral dihydrocodeine is equivalent to 10 mg of morphine or 6 mg of diamorphine given by CSCI.

Fentanyl

Fentanyl is very rarely used as a CSCI because the volumes required are large, but there are a few case reports of its use. It is a synthetic opioid, active at the μ-receptor, and is about 75 times more potent than morphine. Equi-analgesic dose ratios are not easy to calculate.

Glycopyrronium

Glycopyrronium is an antimuscarinic used in the treatment of excessive respiratory secretions and bowel colic. It may be used as an alternative to hyoscine hydrobromide for managing terminal secretions because it is cheaper, more potent, does not cross the blood–brain barrier and causes less risk to the eye in patients with glaucoma. It does not relieve symptoms due to secretions that are already present, so must be used as soon as the excessive secretions begin to develop.

Haloperidol

Haloperidol is an antipsychotic drug that is useful as an anti-emetic and for agitation. It is useful for opioid-induced nausea and vomiting, and for hiccups. Haloperidol is compatible with diamorphine if mixed in the same syringe. It is not particularly sedative at lower doses.

Hydromorphone

Hydromorphone is a semi-synthetic opioid derived from morphine. It is more soluble than morphine and about 7.5 times more potent than morphine. It may cause less nausea, vomiting and constipation than morphine, and it appears to be safer in renal failure.

Note: Hydromorphone is not compatible with hyaluronidase, which may be used to reduce inflammation at the injection site.

Hyoscine butylbromide (do not confuse with hyoscine hydrobromide)

Hyoscine butylbromide is useful for bowel colic associated with obstruction, and for excessive bronchial secretions (hyoscine hydrobromide is more effective for bronchial secretions). It causes a dry mouth, retention of urine and constipation. As it does not cross the blood–brain barrier, it does not cause sedation. Usual doses are 60–180 mg per 24 hours.

Hyoscine hydrobromide (do not confuse with hyoscine butylbromide)

Hyoscine hydrobromide is useful for bronchial secretions, colic associated with obstruction, and nausea, and it is also sedative. Usual doses are 800–2400 mg per 24 hours.

Ketamine

Ketamine is a general anaesthetic which, at sub-anaesthetic doses, offers analgesia with minimal sedation. No controlled trials are available, and all reports of its use as an analgesic are based on case studies. It may relieve allodynia and hyperalgesia, but can cause confusion, delirium, hallucinations, hypertension, nightmares and tachycardia. It can interact with opioids, and this can result in opioid toxicity.

Ketorolac

Ketorolac is an NSAID with strong analgesic activity. It should only be used for bone pain when other NSAIDs are ineffective or impractical. A proton pump inhibitor must be prescribed to protect the gastric mucosa. The opioid dose should be reduced, other NSAIDs must be discontinued, and it must be used with extreme caution in liver and renal disease or where there is any risk of gastrointestinal bleeding.

Levomepromazine

Levomepromazine is a broad-spectrum, sedative anti-emetic which is useful for agitation and also for nausea, but local irritation at the injection site is possible. It has a long half-life and this can result in sedation, which might be an unwanted effect.

Methadone

Methadone is a synthetic opioid which is active at the δ- and μ-receptors and is metabolised in the liver. It has a long half-life of over 30 hours and a variable but high bioavailability, making dosing very individual and difficult to predict. It can cause severe irritation at the injection site. Several drugs, including anticonvulsants and monoamine oxidase inhibitors (MAOIs), interact with methadone.

Metoclopramide

Metoclopramide is a non-sedating anti-emetic and prokinetic and therefore is useful for vomiting induced by drugs, gastric stasis and partial outflow obstructions, but it must not be used in patients with complete obstruction of the bowel.

Midazolam

Midazolam is a short-acting benzodiazepine that is useful for anxiety, hiccup, myoclonic jerking, seizures and terminal agitation. Although it is used for hiccup, it can cause this symptom as well. As it is metabolised in the liver, reduced doses may be required in liver disease. Tolerance can develop after a few days of use, necessitating increased doses or a change of medication.

Morphine

Morphine is usually given orally in the UK because of the availability of diamorphine, but it is a suitable alternative for CSCI. Subcutaneous morphine is about twice as potent as oral morphine.

Octreotide

Octreotide is a somatostatin analogue which reduces bowel secretions with excessive diarrhoea as in carcinoid syndrome or in large-volume vomiting. One small controlled trial has demonstrated its use in bowel obstruction. Its stability with other drugs has not been fully established, so if there is any doubt, use a second syringe driver.

Ondansetron

Ondansetron is a selective $5HT_3$ antagonist that is useful for nausea and vomiting associated with upper abdominal radiotherapy and chemotherapy. It may be of value in treating diarrhoea associated with carcinoid syndrome.

Phenobarbital

Phenobarbital is a long-acting barbiturate that may be useful for controlling fits. It is unstable with most other drugs and must therefore be given by a separate syringe driver.

Promethazine

Promethazine is a drug with antihistaminic, antimuscarinic and antidopaminergic properties. It is useful as an anti-emetic for nausea resulting from stimulation of the vomiting centre by head and neck radiotherapy or raised intracranial pressure, and for movement-induced vomiting. It is sedative, causes a dry mouth and can cause agitation at higher doses.

Ranitidine

Ranitidine is an H_2 antagonist which reduces gastric acid output and the volume of gastric secretions. It is not as effective as the proton pump inhibitors for offering gastric protection against NSAIDs.

Tramodol

Tramodol is a synthetic drug with a weak μ-receptor activity. About 90% is excreted by the kidney. It is rarely used in a syringe driver, except perhaps for patients with bone pain who cannot continue oral medication. It is much less potent than morphine, and probably requires doses of about 12 times that of parenteral morphine.

Mixing drugs in the syringe driver

Hyaluronidase is sometimes used to reduce local injection site reactions, and has been mixed safely with the other drugs in the list below. Remember that hydromorphone is not compatible with hyaluronidase.

Diamorphine has been mixed with the individual drugs shown in the table overleaf.

Drug	*Comment*
Cyclizine	Can crystallise at concentrations above 20 mg/ml Moderately irritant to skin
Dexamethasone	Compatible at lower concentrations Discard if the mixture becomes cloudy
Haloperidol	Precipitation occurs at concentrations above 1 mg/ml
Hyoscine butylbromide	Compatible at all doses
Hyoscine hydrobromide	Compatible at all doses
Levomepromazine	Can cause skin irritation
Metoclopramide	Compatible at all doses
Midazolam	Compatible, but less soluble
Octreotide	Compatible
Ranitidine	Is apparently compatible with diamorphine

Three-drug combinations

Some combinations of three drugs have been successfully used, but the risk of incompatibility probably increases with concentration. These drug combinations include the following:

- diamorphine/cyclizine/hyoscine
- diamorphine/levomepromazine/hyoscine
- diamorphine/metoclopramide/dexamethasone
- diamorphine/metoclopramide/midazolam
- diamorphine/midazolam/hyoscine.

The following mixtures are **not** compatible and **should not be used**:

- diamorphine/dexamethasone/cyclizine
- diamorphine/dexamethasone/haloperidol
- diamorphine/dexamethasone/levomepromazine
- diamorphine/dexamethasone/midazolam
- diamorphine/octreotide/hyoscine butylbromide.

E Extra information

Discontinuing a CSCI

You can discontinue a subcutaneous infusion if the original indications for using it resolve.

Think about why the CSCI was set up originally and confirm that the following symptoms have improved and the patient can now resume oral medication:

- bowel obstruction
- confusion or restlessness
- conscious level
- dysphagia
- nausea and vomiting.

Calculate the equivalent dose of oral morphine to be prescribed as immediate-release morphine sulphate solution or tablets to be given 4-hourly, or modified-release morphine tablets given every 12 or 24 hours. The total dose of oral morphine for the 24 hours following discontinuation of subcutaneous infusion is three times the total parenteral diamorphine dose (including breakthrough doses) for the previous 24 hours.

Prescribe any additive drugs orally.

Changes in the use and governance arrangements for controlled drugs (July 2006)

The NHS Clinical Governance Support Team has published new guidance for GPs, outlining recent and anticipated changes to the use and governance arrangements for controlled drugs (CDs). Written by Dr Clare Gerada (FRCGP), the guidance outlines the new responsibilities in the management of CDs affecting GPs in England, Scotland and Wales.

From 7 July changes to the Misuse of Drugs Regulations 2001 gave statutory backing to new arrangements for prescribing, dispensing, record-keeping and destruction of CDs, while legislative changes in inspection and monitoring processes are expected in the Health Act Regulations in the autumn.[2]

References

1 Lee P. Designing a simple help card for use with a syringe driver. *Nurs Times.* 2006; **102:** 31–3.

2 Royal College of General Practitioners. *Guidance on Changes in the Management of Controlled Drugs:* www.cgsupport.nhs.uk/downloads/Primary_Care/Controlled_Drugs_Management_Changes.pdf

Further reading

- Dickman A, Schneider J, Varga J. *The Syringe Driver.* Oxford: Oxford University Press; 2005. (This text gives details of combinations of up to five drugs that have been successfully used in syringe drivers, and includes information about the newer devices.)
- Graham F. Syringe drivers and subcutaneous sites: a review. *Eur J Palliat Care.* 2006; **13:** 138–41.
- Laird B, McNeil L, Ross C. The use of implantable pumps in palliative care. *Eur J Palliat Care.* 2006; **13:** 59–62.
- Perdue C. The syringe driver – an aid to delivering symptom control. *Nurs Times.* 2004; **100:** 32–5.

Part 4

Common symptoms and their management

Chapter 19

Abdominal swelling

> In men, nine out of ten abdominal tumours are malignant; in women, nine out of ten abdominal swellings are the pregnant uterus.
>
> Rutherford Morrison (1853–1939)

Introduction

The healthy adult has about 50 ml of fluid in the abdominal cavity, with a turnover of about 5 ml per hour. The protein content is about 25% of that in the plasma.

Up to 50% of cancer patients will have some ascitic fluid in the abdomen. It is commonly associated with ovarian cancer (35%), and also with breast, lung, endometrial and gastrointestinal tract cancers.

Note: Although the differential diagnoses are discussed, the main focus of this chapter is on malignant ascites.

C Consider

Many of the causes of a distended abdomen can be remembered by listing them under the letter 'F' as follows:

- faeces
- fat
- fibroids
- flatus
- fluid (cyst or ascites)
- fetus
- full bladder.

In addition, one must remember to consider the following:

- hepatomegaly
- intestinal obstruction
- ovarian masses.

A Assess

There are a number of questions that should be asked in order to determine the cause and the impact of the abdominal distension on the patient's quality of life.

- *Abdominal girth*. Has the patient's waist measurement been increasing, or have they noticed that clothing or belts are becoming tighter?
- *Ankles*. Has there been any ankle swelling? Ask about use of previous diuretics for heart failure or any other reason.

- *Breathing.* Has there been any difficulty in breathing, including orthopnoea or dyspnoea?
- *Heartburn.* Increasing heartburn and symptoms of reflux oesophagitis may result from increasing intra-abdominal pressure.
- *Squashed stomach.* The typical symptoms are early satiety and nausea. Are either of these a problem?
- *Weight.* A gain in weight might be due to the accumulation of fluid.

Ask whether there are any other physical or emotional symptoms not listed above that might be due to the ascites, and ascertain the impact of each of these symptoms on the patient's daily living.

Working through the list of causes, consider each in turn and eliminate as many as possible.

- *Faeces.* Check for constipation, and don't forget that an empty ballooned rectum indicates a higher obstruction.
- *Fat.* Most patients with advanced cancer will have evidence of loss of weight, but some will be overweight. Look at the umbilicus. In the obese patient it is usually inverted, which is normal, but it often bulges in the ascitic patient. Tense ascites may produce abdominal hernias.
- *Fibroids.* Think about benign and malignant uterine tumours and investigate appropriately if indicated. If no action will be taken, consider the need for and value of invasive procedures.
- *Flatus.* Look for signs of bowel obstruction and a resonant abdomen on percussion.
- *Fluid (cyst or ascites).* Ovarian cysts can be very large and difficult to distinguish from ascites, which is the other relatively common cause in palliative care. Look for 'shifting dullness' where the resonance of the abdomen alters with the patient positioned on one side and then the other as ascitic fluid trickles to the lower regions.
- *Fetus.* This is unlikely, but not impossible. Younger patients may be pregnant and have a malignancy. Seek appropriate advice from the obstetric team.
- *Full bladder.* Ask about urinary output, and if in doubt, catheterise.
- *Hepatomegaly.* The enlarged liver should be palpable, and an area of dullness to percussion should confirm the extent of enlargement.
- *Intestinal obstruction.* Lack of passage of faeces and flatus and a tympanic note on percussion should point to this cause.
- *Ovarian masses.* Ultrasound might be required to confirm the diagnosis.

An ultrasound scan will confirm the presence of ascites and should show whether there are tumour adhesions resulting in smaller pockets of fluid that might not allow a reasonable amount of fluid to be withdrawn.

If a bowel obstruction is suspected, a CT scan should confirm the diagnosis.

Check serum albumin and urea and electrolyte counts first, and check platelet counts and perform clotting screening, if appropriate, if paracentesis is being considered.

℞ Remedy

Note: This applies to ascites.

The most effective way to reduce malignant ascites is to treat the primary cancer with chemotherapy. This may not be a realistic goal, so other measures must be considered.

Analgesia

This may be sufficient in patients who are bedfast and have a short prognosis.

Diuretics

A combination of a loop diuretic, such as furosemide, and spironolactone should be used. If patients have ankle swelling as well as abdominal swelling, offer a diuretic in preference to paracentesis.

Paracentesis

Patients who have liver secondaries usually respond to diuretics, but paracentesis may be used to provide more rapid relief of symptoms.

Paracentesis should be offered if there is:

- dyspnoea due to upward pressure on the diaphragm
- nausea due to gastric squashing
- pain or tightness due to abdominal stretching.

Practical issues with regard to paracentesis are listed below.

- Infection is a possible but relatively rare complication.
- Leakage may occur at the site of cannulation after the procedure. Use a drainable colostomy bag to collect any fluid that gathers.
- Perforation of the bowel is possible if there is an associated obstruction.
- The volume drawn off is usually 2–4 litres, but up to 12 litres of fluid may be present. Removal of too much fluid (6 litres or more) risks hypovolaemia, and the fluid shift from the circulation into the extracellular fluid can cause shock and collapse. Low serum sodium or albumin levels will exacerbate this effect.

If ascites recurs rapidly, consider intracavitary bleomycin to adhere to the peritoneum, and if anticipated life expectancy allows, consider a peritoneo-venous shunt.

Contraindications to paracentesis are as follows:

- coagulopathies
- infection – systemic or local
- liver or kidney failure
- low serum albumin or sodium levels.

Peritoneo-venous shunts

These consist of a catheter in the peritoneal cavity with a one-way valve that allows drainage into the superior vena cava via one of the jugular veins. They are prone to blockage.

E Extra information

The normal turnover of fluid in the peritoneal cavity is 4–5 ml hourly in a healthy person. It can be 100 ml per hour in malignancy.

Blockages of the sub-diaphragmatic lymphatics by peritoneal deposits, combined with sodium retention, are the main factors contributing to the accumulation of ascites.

Malignant ascites is an exudate with a protein content which is about three-quarters of that in the plasma. The rich protein content makes it an excellent medium for growth of cancer cells and bacteria.

Consider the value of complementary therapies to improve comfort, and don't forget about how body image and sexuality may be affected by having ascites.

Further reading

- Campbell C. Controlling malignant ascites. *Eur J Palliat Care.* 2001; **8:** 187–90.
- Preston N. A review of the management of malignant ascites. *Eur J Palliat Care.* 2005; **12:** 57–60.

Chapter 20

Anorexia and nutrition

> Eat, v.i. To perform successively (and successfully) the functions of mastication, humectation and deglutition.
>
> Ambrose Bierce (1842–1914)[1]

Introduction

Anorexia is a very common symptom, experienced by around 65–85% of cancer patients. Ability to enjoy one's food is one of the most important aspects of a patient's assessment of their quality of life.

C Consider

Serious illnesses like cancer frequently result in reduced physical activity, which in turn results in a decrease in the amount of food required to provide the necessary energy. It is also natural for people who are seriously ill to lose interest in food. The patient may be less worried about this than the relatives and carers.

- *Primary anorexia* is the term used to describe a natural loss of interest in food.
- *Secondary anorexia* is due to some reversible cause.

Why is the patient not eating? Consider each of the following causes:

- altered taste
- constipation
- chemotherapy
- delayed gastric emptying
- denture problems or some other factor making chewing difficult
- depression
- drugs (e.g. antibiotics causing nausea)
- dry or sore mouth
- medications
- metabolic causes (e.g. hypercalcaemia, uraemia)
- nausea or vomiting
- odours in the environment (e.g. the smell of food cooking)
- oral or oesophageal candidiasis
- pain
- peptides produced by the tumour (e.g. tumour necrosis factor, interleukin-1)
- radiotherapy
- squashed stomach syndrome
- swallowing difficulty
- unappetising food
- weakness resulting in inability to cut up food or feed oneself.

There may be more than one cause of anorexia. Each of the reasons identified needs to be addressed and treated if possible.

Find out about the patient's likes and dislikes with regard to food. If possible, try to include foods that they like and can tolerate.

Does the patient like an alcoholic drink? A small aperitif might help, but excessive alcohol consumption suppresses the appetite and leaves less money to spend on food.

A Assess

Take a careful history from the patient to find out the reasons for their loss of appetite. Find out when the problem started and whether it is related to another event, such as starting a particular treatment. Sometimes the cause is very simple, like a poorly fitting denture or some local condition causing pain or difficulty in eating.

An illustrative case history

John was a 48-year-old man who was suffering from a brain tumour which had robbed him of the ability to speak and resulted in weakness of his dominant arm and hand. His inability to cut up his food in order to eat it was misinterpreted as loss of appetite. When he was offered steroids to stimulate his appetite, he shook his head. This was interpreted as refusal of treatment and non-compliance.

Another patient spoke up and explained what John's problem was, and that he was unable to help as he was also bedridden.

A simple observation and assessment would have avoided this inappropriate course of action.

Nutritional assessment

The word 'nutrition' can be used as an aide-memoire as follows.

N	Needing assistance with feeding, cooking or shopping.
U	Unhealthy – appetite affected by disease or treatment.
T	Tooth-related problems – loss of teeth, denture problems or toothache.
R	Reduced social contact – people living alone tend to eat less well.
I	Inappropriate use of available funds or genuine financial problems.
T	Treatment – especially if on three or more types of medication.
I	Involuntary weight loss or gain.
O	Over 75 years of age.
N	Nicotine – speeds up metabolism and suppresses appetite.

The word 'nutrition' can also be used as an aid to assessment of nutritional risk.

	Factor to be assessed	Risk score
N	Needs help with personal care/shopping	2
U	Usually eats less than three meals a day	3
T	Tooth or mouth problems causing difficulty eating	2
R	Regular intake of alcohol of over 3 units daily	2
I	Income problems or inappropriate spending	4
T	Three or more medications daily	1
I	Involuntary weight loss/gain of 6 kg in 6 months	2
O	On their own – no company at mealtimes	1
N	Normal appetite or taste altered due to present illness	2

Add together the scores for each individual factor identified. The risk and the appropriate action to be taken may be identified from the following table.

Score	*Assessment and action*
0–2	Low risk. Reassess at an appropriate time interval according to any changes in circumstances or any perceived risk factor being identified.
3–5	Moderate risk. Advise and modify any factors that can be changed. The patient would benefit from referral to a dietitian.
≥6	High risk. Immediate referral to dietitian advised.

On examining the patient, look for signs of malnutrition such as red tongue, stomatitis, bleeding gums and atrophic skin.

Oesophageal thrush may be present even if the mouth is clean. If this is suspected, treat with a systemic antifungal, as the contact agents such as nystatin are less effective.

Check blood sugar, urea and electrolytes, calcium and serum proteins, and treat any abnormality detected.

℞ Remedy

Identify and treat all reversible causes of the anorexia. If a particular drug appears to be responsible, modify the drug regimen if possible to overcome the problem.

Advise on appropriate dietary measures, taking into account preferred flavours, consistency and quantity of food. Weakness may make it difficult for the patient to cut up their food, and mincing or cutting up food for the patient may be all that is required. This is not anorexia per se, but it is easily overlooked and easily remedied.

Advise the patient and relatives that small regular meals, served on a smaller plate, can be more appealing than a bigger portion which may be returned largely uneaten. High-calorie snacks may be easier to manage than normal-sized meals. Supplement drinks can be sipped slowly from the carton, or if this seems too large to the patient, they may be more appealing if frozen and offered as lollipops.

Patients may be nauseated or put off eating by strong cooking smells.

Seek advice from a specialist nutritional support nurse or dietitian. Emphasise the importance of an adequate fluid intake even if the patient is unable to manage a 'balanced' diet.

Consider the use of corticosteroids as appetite stimulants for patients in whom no identifiable or reversible cause can be found:

- prednisolone 15–30 mg daily, or
- dexamethasone 2–4 mg daily, or
- megestrol acetate, at a dose of 80–160 mg daily.

Megestrol acetate can stimulate the appetite and may result in some weight gain. There is some evidence that responses are dose related.[2] Megestrol acetate may offer an advantage over dexamethasone, in that it appears to have fewer side-effects, but it can cause tumour 'flare' in breast cancer.

Review the patient frequently. Offer clear explanations and reassurance to both the patient and the family, recognising that anorexia often causes greater anxiety for the family than for the patient.

E Extra information

Eating can be very exhausting for a weak, debilitated patient. Cutting up food can be much more tiring than one may imagine, and some patients just can't be bothered. Chewing meat can be exhausting, and a soft diet that requires minimal chewing may be tolerated best. In the short term, dietary supplements and enriched drinks may be helpful, but some of the flavours may not be to the patient's liking, and it may be a case of 'trial and error' to find the most acceptable one. Some are better tolerated if served very cold.

Patients can find anorexia depressing, and for the family it can be very distressing trying to provide adequate nutrition for a patient who has no interest in food. In advanced disease, it may not be realistic to achieve a significant improvement in the patient's nutritional state.

Some patients, especially those suffering from oesophageal or oropharyngeal cancer, may require enteral feeding. Many will be fed via a gastrostomy tube and will require the input of a nutrition nurse specialist, but they can often be managed at home.[3]

Percutaneous endoscopic gastrostomy (PEG) tube feeding has the advantages of being cheaper, safer and more physiological than parenteral feeding.[4] Placement of the PEG tube is associated with a small but significant morbidity.

Enteral tube feeding is regarded as a medical treatment, and this raises ethical issues when it is considered that the burdens of continuing outweigh any benefit. It is advisable to discuss this issue with the competent patient before tube placement, especially if a PEG tube is being considered.

When comparing the value of nasogastric tubes and PEG tubes, the following points should be considered.

	Nasogastric tube feeding	*PEG tube feeding*
Complication rate	Low	Moderate
Insertion	Non-invasive	Invasive
Nutritional benefit	Uncertain	Good
Patient acceptability	Poor	Good
Replacement time	About 1 month or less	Several months

Mouth care and oral hygiene are very important aspects of the patient's care. A nasogastric tube is a foreign body, and some minor trauma and infection risk is unavoidable. Dental decay and pathogens in the mouth might be risk factors for developing aspiration pneumonias in patients with dysphagia who require nasogastric tubes.

Some ways to add extra calories, fat and protein to meals are listed below.

- *Butter* added to cooked rice, cooked pasta and vegetables, etc., adds some calories, fats and vitamins.
- *Buttering* toast while it is hot allows more butter to melt into the toast, resulting in extra calories, fats and vitamins.
- *Creamers* (the type usually added to coffee) add calcium, glucose and vegetable fat.
- *Dried milk* added to ordinary milk (one cup per pint) doubles the protein content.
- *Mayonnaise* is fattier and contains more calories than salad dressing.
- *Milk* can be used instead of water to dilute 'condensed' soups.
- *Soured cream or cheese* on potatoes adds calories and fats.
- *Sugar* can be added to cereals, or syrup to porridge, to provide a source of extra energy.
- *Vitamin drops or medicines* may be used to provide extra vitamins. Since cooking or heating destroys many vitamins, the drops are best added after cooking. The taste may be unacceptable to some patients.
- *Whipped cream* contains a large number of calories and is easy to swallow. It can be added to desserts and puddings.

Ice-cream makers are relatively inexpensive. Home-made ice cream contains cream, milk and sugar and, by adding some puréed fruit, one can provide calories, fats and some roughage.

High-calorie and high-protein powders have little discernible taste and can be added to drinks or soft food.

Suggestions for improving the patient's appetite

- *An aperitif* in the form of a small alcoholic drink may help, provided that the alcohol will not interact with any medication which is currently being prescribed. Some cancer patients become intolerant of alcohol and may even experience pain after having a drink.
- *'Eat when you are hungry'* is a very basic idea that works for many patients. Patients' appetites may not be in step with normal family mealtimes, and their appetite may be greatest in the morning and decrease as the day progresses.
- *Exercising* before meals stimulates the appetite if the patient feels fit enough for exercise. Even a few minutes spent sitting in the fresh air can help.
- *Fruit juice or lemonade* can stimulate the appetite.
- *Individual food preferences* are important. Encourage the patient to eat the things they like and enjoy. In an anorexic patient, intake of any food is more important than its nutritional value.
- *Keep food out of sight* between mealtimes. Anorexic patients find that the sight of food can act as a constant reminder of their loss of appetite and make them feel nauseated.

- *Small portions,* attractively served, are more appetising. If the patient is eating out, most restaurants will happily serve small portions on request. Many will also omit or add a particular food on request.
- *Snacks* help to keep up some food intake. Grated cheese, crisps, dried fruit and nuts or yogurt are good choices.

Altered taste and loss of appetite

Chemotherapy and radiotherapy can affect the patient's sense of taste. Women who are suffering from cancer might notice that they experience the same changes in appetite and taste as they did during pregnancy. Similarly, they might experience the same food cravings and intolerances as they had during pregnancy.

If the patient is undergoing treatment that might affect their appetite or their ability to cook food, planning ahead can help. Some of the following suggestions may be of value.

- *Cold food* has less taste than warm food. Salads and other cold meals can be quite nutritious.
- *Herbal teas* can be acceptable and pleasant, taken hot or cold.
- *Mints and boiled sweets* may help to overcome a bad taste in the mouth. Remind the patient of the risk of dental decay and the fact that hard sweets can cut and ulcerate their tongue and mouth, especially if their mouth is dry.
- *New flavours* are worth a try. Sometimes bland foods become better tolerated, especially during treatment. Radiotherapy that affects the head and neck can cause a sore mouth, and sometimes very bland food is easiest to eat. Some types of chemotherapy can also cause a sore mouth, and strong flavours and spicy foods can sting. If avoidance of food means less discomfort, this may be the cause of the 'anorexia'!
- *Planning ahead.* Before starting a particularly tiring session of treatments, encourage the patient to make and freeze single-portion meals, ready to be used when they feel unable to cope with cooking. Alternatively, a stock of 'convenience foods' and frozen meals might be preferable if cooking is a problem.
- *Plastic utensils* can help to overcome the metallic taste associated with some chemotherapy drugs. Using a normal metal fork or spoon can exacerbate this problem.
- *Sauces and marinades* can add moistness and flavour, both of which are lost in patients who have a dry mouth. Bland flavours may be better tolerated by patients with a sore mouth.
- *Spices* can be added to disguise tastes that are poorly tolerated, but the patient might be more than usually sensitive to spicy foods, and might burn their tongue.

References

1 Bierce A. *The Devil's Dictionary.* Ware: Wordsworth Editions Ltd; 1911.

2 Twycross R, Wilcock A, Charlesworth S *et al. Palliative Care Formulary.* 2nd ed. Oxford: Radcliffe Medical Press; 2002. p. 234.

3 Russell C. The needs of patients requiring home enteral tube feeding. *Prof Nurse.* 2002; **17:** 500–2.
4 Keeley P. Feeding tubes in palliative care. *Eur J Palliat Care.* 2002; **9:** 229–31.

Further reading

- Antoun S. Artificial nutrition at the end of life: is it justified? *Eur J Palliat Care.* 2006; **13:** 194–7.
- Burucoa B, Bely H. Is there still any pleasure in eating for palliative care patients? *Eur J Palliat Care.* 2004; **11:** 60–64.
- Ede S. Artificial hydration and nutrition at the end of life. *Eur J Palliat Care.* 2000; **7:** 210–12.
- Etherlands E. Assessment and management of eating skills in the older patient. *Prof Nurse.* 2004; **19:** 318–22.
- Langlands S, Forbes A. Provision and management of home parenteral nutrition. *Prescriber.* 2004; **15:** 30–44.
- Madigan S. Enteral tube feeding in primary care. *Forum.* 2002; **19:** 32.
- Power J. Nutritional issues in advanced cancer. *Eur J Palliat Care.* 1999; **6:** 39–42.
- Thoresen L, de Soysa AK. The nutritional aspects of palliative care. *Eur J Palliat Care.* 2006; **13:** 190–93.

Chapter 21

Bowel obstruction

> Never let the sun set or rise on a small bowel obstruction.
>
> P Mucha[1]

Introduction

Bowel obstruction occurs most commonly in association with colorectal and ovarian tumours, but can occur in any patient with an abdominal or pelvic cancer.

Obstructions may result from tumours arising in the internal lumen of the bowel, the bowel wall or outside the bowel when the tumour is on the surrounding peritoneum. In many cases the obstruction may occur at multiple levels. Often the clinical presentation is that of obstruction without any evidence of a lesion in the bowel. This is known as a 'functional obstruction.'

Causes of bowel obstruction include the following:

- the original tumour (65% of cases)
- non-malignant causes (e.g. adhesions) (25% of cases)
- a new primary tumour (10% of cases).

C Consider

Does the patient have advanced peritoneal disease? If so, the most likely cause of the obstruction is malignant tumour, although adhesions are a possible cause.

Is this a true obstruction or severe constipation? A plain abdominal X-ray may help to exclude this cause. When thinking about constipation, check the following details.

- Has an opioid been prescribed without a laxative?
- Has there been poor compliance with the laxative prescribed?
- Is the patient unable or reluctant to use the toilet? This may be due to immobility, embarrassment, lack of privacy, rectal pain or tenesmus.

A Assess

Since the management of intestinal obstruction depends on the precise cause, a thorough assessment is vital.

Ask about the patient's bowel habit, concentrating on any recent changes. What is their normal bowel habit? When did it change? Does this change coincide with a change in medications prescribed, such as starting on opioids or increasing the opioid dose without prescribing adequate doses of laxatives?

Make sure that you understand what the patient means when they use words like 'constipation'.

Common signs and symptoms of obstruction include the following:

- constipation or reduced frequency of bowel movements with no flatus passed
- diarrhoea, in the early stage, as liquefying faeces bypass an incomplete blockage

- distension of the abdomen, but be aware that this sign may be absent
- pain which is colicky at first, varying in frequency and intensity but becoming continuous
- vomiting, usually large volumes, often without nausea, and consisting of ingested fluids, saliva and normal bowel secretions or faeces.

On examining the patient, look for the following:

- abdominal distension
- increased bowel sounds
- faecal impaction higher up the rectum (check for ballooning in an empty rectum).

A plain erect and supine abdominal X-ray may reveal fluid levels and help to distinguish between severe constipation and a mechanical obstruction. A CT scan of the abdomen and pelvis might help to detect recurrent tumour.

Is the patient fit for surgery?

℞ Remedy

If a malignant obstruction is diagnosed, what treatment options are appropriate?

If the patient is sufficiently fit, ask for a surgical opinion and an assessment of the advantages and disadvantages of surgery. It is essential to weigh up the mortality and morbidity of surgery against quality of life and the expected prognosis.

Bowel wall oedema

Although firm evidence is not available, a trial of dexamethasone is worthwhile. Start with 8–16 mg subcutaneously (SC) in the mornings. If, after a 3-day trial, the vomiting has subsided, continue with oral steroids. Whether the vomiting would have resolved spontaneously or not will never be known. If there is no response after 3 days, stop the dexamethasone.

Incomplete obstructions and gut motility disorders

Prokinetics such as metoclopramide and domperidone must not be used in complete obstructions, but incomplete obstructions may be relieved by metoclopramide starting with a dose of 30 mg SC per 24 hours.

High-level obstructions might respond to a trial of subcutaneous metoclopramide, 60 mg over 24 hours.

Complete obstruction

In cases of complete obstruction, or where a suspected incomplete obstruction does not resolve with the above regime, the focus must be on symptom management.

Colic

Hyoscine butylbromide, starting with 40 mg per 24 hours, should be given by syringe driver.

Constipation

Having ensured that the obstruction is not caused or worsened by constipation, rectal suppositories or docusate enemas might be helpful. Excessive doses of stimulants should be avoided in order to prevent aggravation of the obstruction.

Nausea and vomiting

Avoid prokinetics. Try cyclizine 100–150 mg per 24 hours via a syringe driver. If this is not sufficient, consider adding levomepromazine 6.25–25 mg per 24 hours via a syringe driver, bearing in mind that this drug may cause drowsiness. Haloperidol 3–5 mg per 24 hours is a useful alternative.

Persistent vomiting might respond to subcutaneous octreotide, a somatostatin analogue which reduces gastrointestinal secretions. The dose should be in the range 300–600 μg per 24 hours. Start with the lower dose and titrate upwards depending on the response.

Nasogastric tube

This is rarely a useful long-term solution to the problem of a bowel obstruction. It is distressing and, as a single measure, it only works in about 20% of patients. If vomiting is not subsiding in response to medical treatment, it might be worth considering.

Nasogastric intubation has several disadvantages.

- It forms a barrier between patient and relative.
- There is a risk of aspiration.
- It can cause undue discomfort.

There will be occasions when the patient finds it preferable to suffer the vomiting. Always discuss with the patient what their choice is, and emphasise that they are allowed to reconsider their choice later, especially if other treatments are working.

E Extra information

Symptoms often begin intermittently and become worse with time as the obstruction worsens. In some cases the obstruction occurs at multiple levels, so patients may not present with all of the classical symptoms listed above. Intestinal obstruction should be considered in all patients with advanced malignancy who are vomiting.

Patients with an obstruction low in the bowel might be able to continue to drink and even to eat small amounts. Sufficient fluid will be absorbed to prevent complete dehydration. It is important to explain this to the patient and their relatives.

Careful attention should be paid to mouth care. Small amounts of moisture will be absorbed through the oral mucosa. This is something the relatives can do that allows them to be usefully involved in the patient's care, and which provides comfort and a small amount of fluid to the patient.

If pain is a problem and requires a subcutaneous infusion of diamorphine, the reduction in gut motility due to the opioid is not a reason for concern at this stage.

Even though life expectancy remains very short, one should aim to enhance quality of life by good symptom control. Simple measures, such as an ice cube to suck or regular mouth care, should be offered. Encourage the family to be involved in these measures.

The family should be offered full support and should be made fully aware of why a more active approach is considered inappropriate.

Reference

1 Mucha P Jr. Small intestinal obstruction. *Surg Clin North Am.* 1987; **67:** 597–620.

Further reading

- Rawlinson F. Malignant bowel obstruction. *Eur J Palliat Care.* 2001; **8:** 142–6.

Chapter 22

Breathlessness

Breathing is the greatest pleasure in life.
Giovanni Papini (1881–1956), Italian author and philosopher

Introduction

Breathlessness is a common symptom among cancer patients, with a prevalence of around 40%.

Dyspnoea must be one of the worst symptoms anyone can suffer. Patients will vary in how they cope. Some will have suffered from chronic obstructive pulmonary disease (COPD) for years and merely experience a worsening of their usual symptoms and be less affected than other patients who have never previously been dyspnoeic.

The sensation of being unable to breathe adequately will generate tremendous panic, and fear of imminent death during a bad attack of breathlessness. The patient and their relatives will be very anxious and frightened. Reassurance and psychological support are essential.

C Consider

Breathlessness in the cancer patient has many possible causes. It is important to identify all of the causes and to deal with each of them. Non-malignant causes of dyspnoea may coexist with the cancer and should not be overlooked because a new disease is present.

Possible causes, some of which are easily reversible, include the following:

- anaemia
- anxiety
- ascites causing pressure on the chest cavity
- bronchospasm
- carcinoma of the bronchus
- cardiac arrhythmias
- COPD
- diaphragmatic weakness
- heart failure
- lung fibrosis
- lymphadenopathy
- lymphangitis carcinomatosa
- mesothelioma
- pericardial effusion
- pleural effusion
- pneumothorax (spontaneous, or secondary to disease or lung biopsy, etc.)
- respiratory muscle weakness
- secondary cancer deposits
- superior vena cava obstruction
- uraemia.

A Assess

Identify and assess the concern felt by the patient and the relatives and their expectations of what is going to happen during a breathless attack. They probably fear that they will die as a result of choking or simply being unable to breathe at all. Both are unlikely, but they are very real concerns and must not be underestimated.

Take a full respiratory history, including the following:

- breathlessness – when it started and how it is changing with time
- cough – when it started and what it is like, dry, or associated with sputum or blood
- haemoptysis – whether it is spots of blood, globules or frank bleeding
- pleuritic pain
- sputum colour and volume.

Acknowledge the fear associated with breathlessness and address the patient's fears associated with suffocation and dying during an attack of dyspnoea. These are real fears and must not be overlooked or underestimated, even though the chances of such an event happening may be small.

Examine the patient, paying attention to the following:

- blood pressure and pulse
- cyanosis – is it peripheral or central?
- dependent oedema
- finger clubbing
- heart rate and rhythm
- respiratory rate and pattern of breathing.

These are all important in identifying the cause.

A plain chest X-ray will confirm the presence of a pleural effusion, but will not always distinguish between an effusion and consolidation. If there is uncertainty, an ultrasound scan should confirm the diagnosis.

Assess the patient's ability to walk and climb stairs, and the impact that breathlessness has on the activities of normal daily life. Be sensitive to the fact that such a loss of independence can be associated with understandable anxiety and depression. How will the patient manage at home? Who is available to help?

Discuss the effects of the illness now and how it might progress, and explore what help is available or might be required as disease progresses and symptoms worsen.

℞ Remedy

Relevant physiology and pathology

The pathophysiology of breathlessness is complex and not fully understood.

Normal respiratory function is under the control of regular activity in the respiratory centre located in the brainstem. Inputs to the respiratory centre include the signals generated in the mechanical stretch receptors in the airways, lung tissue, diaphragm and intercostal muscles.

In addition, the chemoreceptors in the aortic arch, carotid body and medulla monitor the levels of oxygen and carbon dioxide and feed information to the respiratory centre.

Because there are two sets of impulses controlling breathing, distortion or stimulation of the mechanical stretch receptors by lung cancer can produce the sensation of breathlessness even though the blood gas levels are normal. In addition, muscle weakness, fatigue, damage to the phrenic nerve or a restrictive tumour such as mesothelioma can all cause or worsen the sensation of breathlessness.

Non-pharmacological management of breathlessness

These measures should be offered to all breathless patients.

Patients should be offered help to relax. A fan blowing cool air near the face, or encouraging the patient to sit near an open window can help. Physiotherapy, including breathing exercises, is helpful, and patients should be offered drugs to help them to relax and feel more in control by reducing their awareness of breathing if necessary.

Positioning of the patient is important. By sitting upright, the abdominal contents go down, thus taking pressure off the diaphragm and assisting lung expansion. Good positioning also aids relaxation of the upper chest muscles.

Aspiration of excessive secretions is less likely to occur if the patient lies on one side, well propped up.

Drainage of a large pleural effusion will quickly relieve symptoms and can be repeated. This can be performed as an outpatient procedure. Consider pleurodesis for recurrent effusions.

A pleural effusion that is large enough to cause symptoms will be detectable clinically. Aspiration of 500 ml will give relief, but on occasion a larger volume may be safely withdrawn.

Complications of the procedure include haemothorax and pneumothorax.

Pharmacological management of breathlessness

Benzodiazepines

Fears of suffocation or dying during a breathless attack are very real and need to be addressed. The patient may be hyperventilating due to panic.

Diazepam is the usual choice, a dose of 2–5 mg being given twice daily or as required.

Lorazepam and midazolam have shorter half-lives than diazepam and are useful for dealing with emergency situations, but can be associated with reactive anxiety, as their effects wear off relatively quickly.

Bronchodilators

Bronchoconstriction may be present even without obvious wheeze, so it is worth trying a bronchodilator such as nebulised salbutamol or ipratropium.

Cannabinoids

Nabilone at a dose of 0.1–0.2 mg orally four times daily may be helpful for breathless and anxious patients. Higher doses cause drowsiness, and the drug cannot be used if there is atrial fibrillation or heart failure.

Corticosteroids

Corticosteroids probably reduce oedema associated with tumours, and may help in cases of metastases, lymphangitis carcinomatosa and superior vena cava obstruction. Dexamethasone, 4–8 mg once daily, is the treatment of choice and should be discontinued if there is no improvement after several days.

Diuretics

These should be prescribed for cardiac failure.

Opioids

Morphine reduces the excessive respiratory drive associated with hypoxia and hypercapnia. The respiratory rate is reduced, breathing is more efficient and the sensation of breathlessness improves.

Morphine does not cause carbon dioxide retention if prescribed appropriately, and does not cause significant respiratory depression when prescribed properly. Start with 2.5 mg of immediate-release morphine orally, and repeat 4-hourly if it is effective. Modified-release preparations are less effective, and nebulised morphine offers no advantage over the oral medication.

Opioids cause constipation, so always prescribe a laxative at the same time.

Oxygen

Oxygen may help breathlessness in patients with a low PaO_2 at rest or on exertion. Many cancer patients do not have a low enough PaO_2 to gain any physiological benefit from oxygen therapy. Use of oxygen may cause psychological dependence, and is best avoided because of the restrictions on activity and the barrier that oxygen administration can create between the patient and their family.

Saline

Normal saline administered via a nebuliser may help to loosen sticky secretions.

Theophyllines

Theophyllines can improve the sensation of breathlessness even if bronchodilator action is absent.

The half-life of theophylline may be increased in liver and heart failure or by interaction with cimetidine or some antibiotics. The half-life is reduced in heavy smokers and by interaction with certain anticonvulsants.

Reversible causes of breathlessness should be treated appropriately. Some common causes of breathlessness and treatments available are listed in the table below.

Cause of dyspnoea	*Treatment*
Airway obstruction (large airway)	Brachytherapy, corticosteroids, laser therapy
Anaemia	Iron, blood transfusion, erythropoietin
Bronchospasm	Bronchodilators or possibly corticosteroids
Infection	Antibiotics
Lung tumour	Chemotherapy or radiotherapy
Lymphangitis carcinomatosa	Corticosteroids, bronchodilators, possibly diuretics
Pleural effusion	Pleural tap – consider pleurodesis if recurrent
Superior vena cava obstruction	Radiotherapy

E Extra Information

In addition to the above measures, patients need to be taught how to cope with their dyspnoea in the most effective way possible. A three-point plan (ABC) can be adopted, looking at the following points.

Anxiety management

Being tense and anxious will make dyspnoea worse. Relaxation and distraction techniques should be taught and practised.

Breathing effectively

The patient is probably using the upper respiratory accessory muscles of respiration, and needs to learn how to use the diaphragm by pursing the lips to slow exhalation and increase tidal volume, and to use the lower respiratory muscles to breathe more efficiently.

Conservation of energy

The patient must learn to prioritise and focus on the most important activities of daily living. As they learn to breathe more efficiently, realistic new goals can be set. In addition, simple advice can help.

Chairs can be placed in helpful places, such as at the top and bottom of the stairs or midway to the bathroom, to 'break the journey'.

Encourage the patient to sit down when washing and showering. A shower or bath seat may be supplied by the occupational therapist.

Relatives also find breathlessness very worrying to observe, and they should be included in discussions and be aware of the treatment plan if the patient agrees to this.

As a general rule, breathlessness on exertion is more likely to be helped by non-pharmacological interventions, shortness of breath due to cancer may be helped by drugs, and breathlessness at rest may respond to both pharmacological and non-pharmacological measures.

Further reading

- Bhatnagar S, Madhurima S, Mishra S. Dyspnoea in cancer patients. *Eur J Palliat Care.* 2006; **13:** 142–6.
- Estfan B, Walsh D. Opioids and the control of breathing: what do we know? *Eur J Palliat Care.* 2006; **13:** 50–53.
- Filshie J. Acupuncture in palliative care. *Eur J Palliat Care.* 2000; **7:** 41–4.
- Rawlinson F. Dyspnoea and cough. *Eur J Palliat Care.* 2001; **7:** 161–4.
- Shee C. End-stage respiratory failure. *Eur J Palliat Care.* 2003; **10:** 98–101.

Chapter 23

Cachexia

> I am no better in mind than in body; both alike are sick and I suffer double hurt.
>
> Ovid (43 BC – AD 17) *Tristia* III, viii, 33

Introduction

Cachexia is a word derived from two Greek words, *kakos* (bad) and *hexis* (condition).

The condition affects up to 80% of cancer patients, is distressing to the patient because the weight loss causes serious changes in body image, and distresses the relatives, who encourage the patient to eat more, but with no resulting weight gain.

Cachexia is a complex mix of symptoms comprising the following:

- anaemia
- anorexia
- organ dysfunction
- reduced appetite and feeling full
- wasting of muscles
- weakness
- weight loss.

Cachexia is more common in solid tumours of the lung, gut and pancreas, but less common in breast cancer. With the exception of breast cancer, the size of the tumour and the amount of weight lost do not seem to be correlated.

C Consider

There are a number of causes of cancer cachexia, including the following:

- decreased nutritional intake
- increased nutritional losses
- metabolic changes
- poor appetite or poor eating habits
- psychological problems, including depression, resulting in failure to look after oneself
- treatment side-effects.

Decreased nutritional intake

This is probably the most important issue. It has several causes, including the following:

- anorexia
- dysphagia

- bowel obstruction resulting in decreased nutritional intake
- malabsorption.

Increased nutritional losses

- Blood loss.
- Diarrhoea and protein loss via the intestines.

Metabolic changes

- Abnormal metabolism mimicking insulin resistance with increased energy expenditure unrelated to the extent of disease.
- Altered carbohydrate metabolism.
- Altered lipid metabolism.
- Altered protein metabolism.

Treatment side-effects

- Chemotherapy may be associated with nausea, vomiting or mucositis, thus reducing food intake.
- Radiotherapy can cause anorexia, nausea, vomiting, diarrhoea and a dry or sore mouth.

A Assess

Find out how much weight has been lost in the previous 3 months. A loss of 10% or more of body weight constitutes malnutrition.

Ask about possible reasons for poor food intake and, if necessary, use the assessment tool in Chapter 20 on anorexia and nutrition (*see* page 94).

Look at the skin to see whether it is dry and scaly.

Look at the mouth to see whether there is stomatitis, cheilosis or glossitis, indicating iron and vitamin deficiencies.

Assess muscle bulk and muscle strength.

Look for pitting oedema.

℞ Remedy

If any of the reasons for poor food intake are reversible, these should be addressed now.

The most effective remedy is to control the tumour growth. However, this may not be a realistic goal.

Ask the dietitian about food supplements, speak to the occupational therapist about ways to make daily life easier, and arrange appropriate physiotherapy.

Steroids may stimulate the appetite but they do not increase muscle mass. Any weight gain is possibly due to fluid retention. The feeling of well-being associated with steroids may be of psychological value.

Progestogens such as megestrol acetate 160–320 mg daily may improve appetite, but can take up to 2 weeks to start to act.

One study found that nutritional supplements combined with an omega-3 fatty acid can halt weight loss and even result in weight gain.[1]

E Extra information

Malignant tumours produce a variety of cytokines, including tumour necrosis factor, interleukins and other agents that break down proteins and fat and cause serious metabolic disturbances.

The ability to tolerate and respond to treatment is much reduced in the cachectic patient.

There is no evidence that total parenteral nutrition prolongs the patient's life.

References

1 Anon. EPA supplement benefit in cancer cachexia. *Prescriber.* 2002; **13:** 13.

Further reading

- Burucoa B, Bely H. Is there still any pleasure in eating for palliative care patients? *Eur J Palliat Care.* 2004; **11:** 60–64.
- Langlands S, Forbes A. Provision and management of home parenteral nutrition. *Prescriber.* 2004; **15:** 30–44.
- Power J. Nutritional issues in advanced cancer. *Eur J Palliat Care.* 1999; **6:** 39–42.

Chapter 24

Confusion

> In a disordered mind, as in a disordered body, soundness of health is impossible.
>
> Cicero (106–43 BC), *Tusculanarum Disputationum,* Book III

Introduction

Stedman's electronic medical dictionary[1] offers the following definitions.

- *Confusion* is a mental state in which reactions to environmental stimuli are inappropriate because the person is bewildered, perplexed or unable to orientate him- or herself.
- *Delirium* is an altered state of consciousness, consisting of confusion, distractibility, disorientation, disordered thinking and memory, defective perception (illusions and hallucinations), prominent hyperactivity, agitation and autonomic nervous system overactivity, caused by a number of toxic structural and metabolic disorders.
- *Terminal agitation* is a combination of delirium and extreme anxiety sometimes seen in the last days of life.

Confusion is usually a manifestation of an organic disorder of one or more causes. It often presents as forgetfulness and may be exacerbated by being in a strange environment. Impaired hearing and sight compound the problem. Neglect of personal care is commonly seen, and the patient may be noisy, aggressive and demanding.

Confusional states and delirium are usually reversible, but there might not be time for improvement in a terminally ill patient. Multiple organ failure can cause delirium and is irreversible.

C Consider

Possible causes of confusion include the following:

- Alzheimer's disease
- anxiety and depression
- brain tumours – primary or secondary
- constipation
- drugs, including alcohol withdrawal, benzodiazepines (or benzodiazepine withdrawal), digoxin, nicotine withdrawal, opioids, selective serontonin reuptake inhibitor (SSRI) withdrawal, steroids (or steroid withdrawal). Opioids accumulate in uraemia, and benzodiazepines and phenothiazines accumulate in liver failure
- hypercalcaemia
- hypoglycaemia
- hyponatraemia due to the syndrome of inappropriate antidiuresis (SIAD) causing water retention with concentrated urine
- hypoxia

- infections
- liver failure
- renal failure
- stroke or transient ischaemic attack (TIA).

Confusion often has more than one cause, and this should be kept in mind. Pain and urinary retention may exacerbate the problem, but the patient may not be able to report these symptoms.

A Assess

Determining the patient's previous mental state and what may be causing confusion will help to clarify the treatment options and possible outcomes of treatment. Without this understanding, it is not possible for a team of carers to manage the problem effectively or to help the patient's family.

Often the family will be able to provide the most accurate account of the patient's recent mental state.

A full clinical examination is essential.

An examination of the mental state should also be undertaken to assess the following:

- orientation in time and place
- memory – for example, asking the patient to remember a name and address
- ability to calculate simple sums
- attention span by the 'serial sevens', where the patient starts at 100 and repeatedly subtracts the number 7 from the previous score
- ability to recognise common objects.

Carry out biochemical assessment to check liver and renal function, corrected calcium and blood sugar levels. The cause is probably multi-factorial, so these results alone might not reveal the full clinical picture.

In practice, confusion in terminally ill patients is often due to a combination of factors, with some reversible features and some residual deficit in brain function.

Assess the risk of self-harm and the risk to other patients.

℞ Remedy

Treat any identifiable causes that can be alleviated. Confusion may be the result of correctly identified but incorrectly interpreted external stimuli. Explanation and reassurance should always be offered, and may be all that are needed.

Make sure that there is adequate light. Try to ensure a quiet calm atmosphere and, as far as possible, ensure that family members, or staff who are known to the patient, care for him or her.

Prevent the patient from harming him- or herself and others.

Drugs should only be used when absolutely necessary.

Night sedation should not be offered routinely. Try to deal with possible causes of insomnia by addressing pain, reducing fear and anxiety and ensuring as quiet an environment as possible. Check that steroids are given early in the day.

If necessary, consider the use of haloperidol, but levomepromazine may be used and is more sedating. Most antipsychotic drugs lower the threshold for convulsions, and this risk must be considered in patients who are susceptible to fitting.

The medication that is offered should reflect the patient's presenting symptoms.

Confused and drowsy

Sedation is not necessary, so choose a non-sedating antipsychotic such as haloperidol 1.5–3 mg at night or risperidone 0.5–1.0 mg twice daily. In the elderly patient, these doses should be halved initially until one establishes the dose required. Risperidone should be avoided in patients with a history of cardiovascular disease.

Confused and agitated

A sedative antipsychotic such as levomepromazine, 25–50 mg orally or via a syringe driver, or chlorpromazine 25–50 mg twice daily orally are reasonable choices for this situation. Reduced doses should be used in the older patient.

Confused and aggressive

These patients are acutely disturbed, may become violent and can represent a danger to themselves and others. Parenteral drugs are essential and should be rapidly acting.

Try haloperidol, 5 mg SC or IM, either alone or combined with lorazepam 1–2 mg SC or IM, and repeat after 30 minutes if necessary. These doses should be halved in the elderly patient.

Alcohol withdrawal

If this is thought to be the cause of confusion, the best treatment in the palliative care setting is to allow the patient to have measured amounts of alcohol, provided that they can swallow.

Clomethiazole, alone or in combination with a benzodiazepine, is the usual drug treatment.

Wernicke's encephalopathy is a possible diagnosis if the patient develops any of the following:

- acute confusion (not alcohol induced)
- ataxia (not alcohol induced)
- loss of consciousness or coma (not alcohol induced)
- memory disturbance
- nystagmus
- seizures.

Wernicke's encephalopathy is caused by a deficiency of thiamine and should be treated with high-potency parenteral B-complex vitamins. The diagnosis is confirmed by checking the red blood cell transketolase levels.

E Extra information

As the time of death approaches, ideally there is an opportunity for reconciliation between the patient and their family, a time for healing rifts, strengthening relationships and saying the final goodbye.

If the dying person is confused, this time may lose its meaning. It can become instead a time of great anguish and distress, not only for the patient but also for the family and those involved in care. Families may carry disturbing memories of their confused relative with them into bereavement, and this may influence their ability to cope with life and loss in the future.

Sensitivity is required as family members are unable to have meaningful conversations with the patient. They may express guilt that they 'left it too late' to say something important.

Although some confused patients clearly have insight and are in a position to be involved in treatment decisions, most do not. The caring team and the patient's family must together decide the best treatment options. Sometimes this can involve sedating a patient who is already quite frail, with the known risk that they may then develop a chest infection by virtue of inactivity and not being able to sit up and cough adequately. The family should be made aware of the reasons for these decisions and be allowed to participate in honest discussion about the issue of sedation.

Further reading

- Anderson T, Watson M, Marr K. Serotonin syndrome: a hidden danger in palliative care. *Eur J Palliat Care.* 2005; **12:** 97–100.
- Burgess L. Addressing the palliative care needs of people with dementia. *Nurs Times.* 2004; **100:** 36–9.
- George J, Lee S. Delirium in terminal illness. *Eur J Palliat Care.* 2005; **12:** 185–7.
- Power D. Terminal care in dementing illness. *Forum. 2005;* **May issue:** 45–6.

Chapter 25

Constipation

> The examining physician often hesitates to make the necessary examination because it involves soiling the finger.
>
> William J Mayo (1861–1939)[1]

Introduction

Constipation, in this text, is the term used to describe difficult or painful defaecation which is less frequent than what is normal for the individual patient, and which is associated with harder and smaller stools.

Almost half of all patients admitted to hospices are constipated. Some may present with diarrhoea which is caused by severe constipation with overflow of liquefied faeces above the faecal mass.

Constipation can cause pain, bowel obstruction, retention of urine and diarrhoea. It distresses the patient and should be treated promptly or avoided by the appropriate prescription of laxatives, especially when opioids are prescribed.

C Consider

There are many possible causes of constipation, which fall into the following categories.

Bowel obstruction

Do not overlook the possibility of bowel obstruction. *See* Chapter 21.

Dehydration

- Decreased fluid intake or increased losses due to vomiting or excessive sweating.

Disease related

- Decreased appetite and low residue intake due to anorexia.
- Immobility.

Drugs

- Anticholinergics.
- Diuretics.
- Granisetron and ondansetron.
- Hyoscine, phenothiazines or tricyclic antidepressants.
- Octreotide.
- Opioids – were they prescribed without a laxative?

Immobility and weakness

Various conditions make it difficult to achieve the necessary increase in intra-abdominal pressure for evacuation. These include the following:

- decreased peristalsis associated with immobility
- general debility of cancer
- paraplegia.

Other causes

- Embarrassment about sharing a toilet.
- Inability to get to the toilet unaided.
- Pain on defaecation due to local problem such as haemorrhoids or anal fissure.

Constipation can be the cause of several other symptoms, including the following:

- abdominal pain
- bowel obstruction
- confusion and restlessness
- diarrhoea
- faecal incontinence
- retention of urine.

A Assess

What does the patient understand by the term 'constipation'? Does their definition match your own?

What was their normal pattern of bowel action prior to their illness or to starting medication?

When did the problem start? Was it associated with starting a new medication or a change in the dose of a drug that was already being prescribed?

What laxatives, if any, is the patient currently taking? Find out whether they are actually taking the laxative as prescribed. Some laxatives are very sweet, and patients may be intolerant of the flavour or may feel nauseated and not take the doses prescribed.

Could the constipation be associated with the patient's diet?

Is the patient's fluid intake appropriate? Is there excessive fluid loss through vomiting, sweating or polyuria?

Is the patient too weak or too immobile to reach the toilet? Are the toilet arrangements convenient and appropriate to the needs of the patient?

Is the patient suffering from a malignant tumour of the gut?

Examine the abdomen, looking for distension, tenderness (especially over the caecum) and faecal masses. Faecal masses usually indent on pressure, and will disappear after treating the constipation. A tumour does neither of these things.

A rectal examination should be performed on all constipated patients. Inspection of the anus, prior to a rectal examination, may reveal an obvious painful cause of constipation, such as prolapsed haemorrhoids, an anal fissure or perianal infection.

An empty ballooned rectum indicates a higher obstruction. Overflow of liquid faeces from above this blockage may present as 'diarrhoea'. Plain abdominal X-ray is helpful in confirming the diagnosis.

Check for hypokalaemia and hypercalcaemia.

If the constipation is caused by an operable solitary obstruction in a patient with a suitable prognosis, speak to a surgeon about the surgical options.

℞ Remedy

Relevant physiology and pharmacology

All opioids slow down gut motility. Analgesics containing codeine in small doses are capable of causing severe constipation, but this may be overlooked. This increased bowel transit time allows for increased reabsorption of water from the stool. There is therefore a dual problem consisting of slowed peristalsis and drier, harder bowel content.

When opioids are used, the regular administration of both a bowel stimulant and a faecal softener is essential.

Anticholinergic drugs cause constipation by a direct action on the gut wall, slowing down peristalsis.

The best remedy for constipation is anticipation and appropriate laxative prescribing, especially when prescribing opioids or other drugs that are known to increase the likelihood of constipation and reduced gut motility.

Non-pharmacological management

- Assess bowel function regularly.
- Fibre and fruit intake should be increased if possible.
- Fluid intake should be increased if possible.
- Mobility should be encouraged.
- Toilets should be convenient and private. Assess the need for and provide any aids to independence, such as a raised toilet seat or supports to aid sitting and standing.

Pharmacological management

- Always prescribe prophylactic laxatives when starting opioids or increasing the dose.
- Use a combination of a stimulant laxative and a faecal softener.
- The amounts of softener and stimulant should be adjusted to suit the individual.

Laxatives basically fall into the following categories:

- bulking agents
- faecal softeners
- osmotic agents
- stimulants
- suppositories and enemas.

Bulking agents

The two most commonly used bulking agents are ispaghula husk and methylcellulose. They are not sufficiently powerful to relieve the constipation associated with opioids, and may even make the patient feel full and result in them not wishing to eat.

Faecal softeners

These drugs (e.g. docusate) are usually given in combination with a stimulant laxative to overcome the effect of opioids on gut motility. They are rarely sufficiently effective on their own.

Osmotic agents

This group includes lactulose, the macrogols and magnesium salts.

One of the problems with these drugs is that, in order to be maximally effective, they need to be taken with reasonably large amounts of fluids, and some patients cannot manage this.

Lactulose is sometimes not well tolerated because it tastes very sweet, causes flatulence and can cause abdominal cramping.

Lactitol powder, which has a similar action to lactulose, may be sprinkled on food.

Stimulants

Examples of stimulant laxatives include bisacodyl, dantron and senna.

Dantron is only licensed for prescribing to patients with a terminal illness. It is often combined with softeners such as docusate (co-danthrusate) or poloxamer (co-danthramer). It can colour the urine red and can cause perineal soreness on skin contact.

Do not use stimulant laxatives if an intestinal obstruction is suspected.

Suppositories and enemas

Arachis oil, bisacodyl, glycerol and phosphate are the main agents used.

Arachis oil retention enemas are administered at night and left to act by lubricating and softening the stool.

The arachis oil enema is usually followed with a phosphate enema to stimulate rectal emptying.

Bisacodyl suppositories need to be in contact with the rectal mucosa in order to be absorbed and stimulate evacuation.

Glycerol is a softener and lubricant.

More severe constipation may require manual evacuation. Polyethylene glycol may be given for 3 days and may be helpful in cases of faecal impaction.

If the rectum is filled with hard faecal masses, do not give a faecal expander. This will only convert a small hard mass into a large soft one that is almost impossible to expel.

E Extra information

Constipation makes the patient miserable, and everything should be done to improve their comfort while medications and other interventions are taking effect. Abdominal massage and local heat may provide comfort, even if they do not actually deal with the problem.

Biochemical abnormalities such as hypercalcaemia and hypokalaemia cause constipation. Hypothyroidism and diabetes mellitus may also be contributory factors.

The dose of laxative required is the dose necessary to ensure a bowel action. Constipated patients may require a higher dose initially. To avoid diarrhoea, this is later reduced to a smaller maintenance dose.

In tumours of the bowel that cause a restricted lumen, the stools should be kept as soft as toothpaste. Use laxatives with softening properties, maintain adequate fluid intake and avoid non-digestible foods, fruit peel and pith.

Surgical intervention is the obvious treatment for a single mechanical obstruction. However, it must be borne in mind that a patient with recurrent malignant disease may have multiple sites of obstruction, which would not be amenable to surgical resection. Many patients find the prospect of a colostomy or ileostomy unacceptable. This should be taken into account when surgery is considered.

Further reading

- Mohsen A, Wilkinson M. Current management options for chronic constipation. *Prescriber.* 2005; **16:** 45–52.
- Perdue C. Managing constipation in advanced cancer care. *Nurs Times.* 2005; **101:** 36–40.
- Yiannakou Y, Cowlam S. Management of constipation. *Prescriber.* 2004; **15** (6).

Chapter 26

Cough and haemoptysis

Cough: a convulsion of the lungs, vellicated by some sharp serosity.
Samuel Johnson (1709–1784), *Dictionary of the English Language*

Since these two symptoms are closely related, they are included in the same chapter. Cough is dealt with first, and haemoptysis is discussed later in the chapter.

Introduction

Cough serves to clear the airways of foreign materials or excessive secretions. It is a common symptom that affects about half of all cancer patients and around 80% of lung cancer patients.

One-third of lung cancer patients will have some haemoptysis, but only about two or three in 100 will have a major bleed.

Cough

C Consider

Cough can be divided into two subgroups:

- dry cough
- wet or, more correctly, productive cough.

Common causes of cough include the following:

- airways disease (COPD)
- bronchial invasion by tumour
- cancer of the lung or pleura – either primary or secondary
- drugs (e.g. ACE inhibitors)
- infection
- left heart failure
- oesophageal reflux
- pleural effusion
- sinus infection with post-nasal drip.

A Assess

A careful history and assessment of the symptoms will identify the cause of the cough in the majority of patients. As a quick guide, common symptoms and causes are tabulated opposite.

Symptom	*Likely cause*
Copious frothy pink sputum	Left heart failure
Copious frothy white sputum	Bronchorrhoea associated with alveolar cell lung carcinoma (rare)
Cough worse lying down	Left heart failure Oesophageal reflux
Cough associated with hoarseness	Vocal cord paralysis
Dry cough	ACE inhibitors Asthma Endobronchial cancer Pleural effusion
Haemoptysis	Lung malignancy
Purulent sputum in an afebrile patient	Bronchiectasis Decompensation of COPD
Purulent sputum in a febrile patient	Lung abscess Pneumonia
Stuffy nose and cough	Sinusitis and post-nasal drip

℞ Remedy

Relevant physiology

Cough is the result of chemical or mechanical stimulation of receptors in the respiratory tract with nerve impulses carried to the respiratory muscles and the medulla.

Coughing requires intact and functional abdominal and chest muscles and the strength to use these muscles effectively.

To expel sputum, one must generate a raised intrathoracic pressure. This requires the brief closure of the glottis, which may not be possible if there is paralysis of the vocal cords, which can occur in cancer of the upper left lung. The resultant cough is ineffective, repetitive and exhausting.

Most drugs that depress consciousness suppress the cough reflex.

Pharmacological management of cough

Dry cough

Deal with reversible causes first. Having excluded these, a dry cough should be suppressed, especially in the terminally ill.

Two types of suppressants exist, namely those that act centrally and those that act peripherally.

Centrally acting cough suppressants

Codeine

Codeine can be tried at a dose of 30–60 mg four times daily. Codeine is constipating, so prescribe a laxative and think about the effect of inducing constipation in a patient who may be weak and short of breath already.

Diamorphine

Diamorphine may be administered by subcutaneous infusion at a dose of 5–10 mg over 24 hours. As with all opioids, constipation is an unwanted side-effect and must be anticipated and treated.

Note: In patients who are already on opioids, titrate the dose according to effect, bearing in mind that there is little evidence to support the use of high doses.

Pholcodine

Pholcodine, 10 ml three times daily, is not as sedating as the analgesic opioids, causes less constipation, and should be tried if the patient is not already on opioids.

Peripherally acting cough suppressants

If the patient is terminally ill or the aim is not to aid the expectoration of sputum, blocking the cough receptors in the bronchioles and the carina may be more appropriate.

Bupivicaine 0.25% or lidocaine 0.2% may be given via a nebuliser at a dose of 5 ml three times daily. These agents, being local anaesthetics, will suppress coughing but will also anaesthetise the throat, so eating and drinking must be avoided for 1 hour after administration in order to avoid aspiration of food or drink.

Productive cough

If the patient is well enough to cough and expectorate, the aim is to facilitate effective coughing. In weak, terminally ill patients, this is an inappropriate aim.

Patients who are able to cough effectively

Antibiotics

Chest infections should be treated with an antibiotic. If sputum is difficult to obtain for culture and sensitivity tests, a macrolide antibiotic such as erythromycin is a reasonable choice.

Bronchodilators

Bronchospasm should be treated with nebulised salbutamol.

Carbocysteine

The evidence that carbocysteine reduces the viscosity of mucus is poor, but it does appear to prolong the time between relapses of COPD and lessen the duration of exacerbations.

Nebulised saline

Nebulised saline can be used to loosen tenacious sputum.

Patients who are too weak to cough effectively

Cough suppressants

See the above section on 'dry cough.'

Radiotherapy

A few patients with lung cancer, including alveolar cancer, will develop a syndrome known as 'bronchorrhoea' in which they produce large amounts of clear frothy sputum.

Radiotherapy may help.

It has been noted that haloperidol reduces the antitussive actions of certain opioids. Haloperidol is a potent sigma-ligand, and the antitussive effect is probably mediated at the sigma sites.

Cough linctuses are generally not used, but might occasionally be helpful if given at night to aid sleep. Their value is unproven and their mode of action is uncertain.

Haemoptysis

C Consider

Haemoptysis may be related to the lung cancer itself, or may be associated with any of the following:

- anticoagulants
- clotting disorders (e.g. thrombocytopenia)
- infection
- liver disease with associated clotting defects.

A Assess

The blood could have come from several sources – lung, gut or epistaxis.

Is the patient on a drug that might cause bleeding (e.g. an NSAID)? A patient with lung cancer may have bled from the gut following administration of a gastro-erosive agent.

Is there a relevant history of a gastric ulcer or respiratory disease that could account for the bleed?

Has the patient been treated for episodes of bleeding?

Has the patient been coughing or vomiting small amounts of blood?

Think about the most likely cause of haemoptysis in this patient:

- bleeding from a lung tumour
- clotting disorder or excessive dose of anticoagulants
- infection
- pulmonary embolism.

Check clotting screen and platelet count and check liver function.

℞ Remedy

Exclude and treat infection.

If coughing stimulates the haemoptysis, consider the use of a cough suppressant (e.g. codeine).

Treat any other clotting disorder that is discovered.

Try an oral haemostatic agent (e.g. tranexamic acid) and continue this for 7 days after the bleeding has stopped.

If bleeding recurs after stopping haemostatic agents, restart them and continue them indefinitely.

If there is a known lung tumour, ask the radiotherapist about the use of radiotherapy to seal the vessel. Usually one fraction is sufficient.

Prepare for sudden massive haemorrhage. Insert a cannula if one is not already in place, and have dark-coloured towels readily available and an anxiolytic to hand for urgent administration. Small bleeds can be the warning sign of a larger bleed later.

Massive haemoptysis

- Position the patient head down to reduce symptoms due to suffocation, which is the usual mode of death in such events. Although it makes *theoretical* sense to position the patient with the affected side down in order to reduce bleeding into the good lung, in practice it rarely makes any difference and possibly causes undue stress to the patient by repositioning them.
- Use dark-coloured towels. Blood looks less obvious on these and it might help to reduce the impact of the amount of blood lost. This is of more benefit to the relatives who may be present or any patients who may witness this distressing event, which may be expected, but the timing is always unpredictable.
- Administer a sedative (e.g. diamorphine 10–30 mg). The intravenous route is fastest, but veins often collapse quickly. Alternatively, give midazolam 5 mg IM. There is no evidence that this does any good, but the relatives will appreciate that everything was done to minimise awareness of the dying patient.

If the possibility of a massive bleed is recognised, it is best to have a frank discussion with the family, and to agree that sedation will be given but that futile attempts at resuscitation will not be undertaken.

E Extra information

Massive haemoptysis is a sudden event and, although it may be expected, it can happen without warning and one can never guarantee that other patients or relatives will not witness the event. It is prudent to sensitively warn relatives about the possibility of a sudden massive haemoptysis. They may feel that they should be by the patient's bedside 24 hours a day. This attitude should be realistically addressed.

Remember that other patients have witnessed a death, and that they also saw how the staff dealt with it. This can either reassure them of the care they can expect or introduce new fears, so be aware of how you deal with these events.

Relatives often express guilt because they were not present at the time of death. Acknowledge the amount of time they have given and the stress they are already experiencing. No one should feel guilty about taking time to eat or sleep.

Further reading

Cough

- Rawlinson F. Dyspnoea and cough. *Eur J Palliat Care.* 2000; **7:** 161–4.
- Zhigniew Z, Krajnik M. The use of antitussives in terminally ill patients. *Eur J Palliat Care.* 2004; **11:** 225–9.

Haemoptysis

- Anwar D, Shaad N, Maxxacato C. Treatment of haemoptysis in palliative care patients. *Eur J Palliat Care.* 2003; **10:** 137–9.

Chapter 27

Depression and sadness

> To run away from trouble is a form of cowardice and, while it is true that the suicide braves death, he does it not for some noble object but to escape some ill.
>
> Aristotle (384–322 BC), *Nicomachean Ethics*

Introduction

The incidence of depression varies from one survey to another, so an exact figure is hard to find, but the average figure seems to be around 25%, although the use of antidepressants in hospices probably does not support this figure.

Certain cancers, including pancreatic cancer, appear to be more strongly associated with depression.[1]

One could argue that the patient's mood lies somewhere on a continuum as follows:

Sadness→→→→Adjusting to the situation→→→→Depression

It is understandable that every patient with any illness may feel sad, angry or bitter and may seem quite 'depressed'. However, it is important to decide which it is and whether the patient is clinically depressed and requires treatment.

Sadness should respond to the opportunity to express one's feelings and the offer of appropriate support. Clinical depression may require specific drug therapy in addition to psychological support.

C Consider

Depressed patients are always sad. Sad patients are not necessarily depressed. Patients with advancing cancer may be understandably sad. As a general rule, if the patient is ill as a result of their sadness, they are probably clinically depressed.

There are some clues to the diagnosis that can be considered before seeing the patient.

- Is there impaired concentration, reduced verbal communication with carers or other patients, and a desire to sit down or lie in bed and not do anything?
- Does the patient have a history of endogenous depression or psychiatric illness?
- Has the patient expressed any thoughts of suicide?
- Is there any family history of depression or psychiatric illness?
- Has there been any recent change in medication to precipitate this event? Steroids can induce depression and psychosis in some patients.
- What is the patient's mood on wakening? The 'depressed' patient tends to feel dreadful at the beginning of the day. In contrast, the 'sad' patient will tend to feel worse as the day goes on and reality draws in again.

A Assess

The diagnosis of depression is made by assessing a number of physical and mental symptoms. It must be remembered that many patients with advanced cancer will be suffering from fatigue and tiredness, may have lost weight and may have altered sleep patterns.

The diagnosis of depression usually involves at least four of the following symptoms being present. To make them easier to recall, I have used the acronym 'IN SAD CASES' that helps me to remember the main areas to assess.

I	Interest lost	no pleasure gained from almost all activities.
N	No 'get up and go'	no interest in or enthusiasm for normal activities.
S	Sleep disturbed	sleeping more or less than usual (due to steroids?)
A	Appetite poor	self-caring patients may have no desire to cook.
D	Dysphoric mood	agitation, restlessness, despondency or despair.
C	Concentration poor	is the newspaper lying untouched?
A	Affect low	feelings of worthlessness – 'Why bother?'
S	Self-reproach	excessive and inappropriate guilt.
E	Energy loss	wanting to lie in bed and do nothing.
S	Suicidal	recurring thoughts about death and suicide.

Reassess the patient daily with respect to the 'five A's':

Activity	are they more or less interested in doing things?
Affect	how has their mood changed since the last assessment?
Anamnesis	has their memory improved or worsened?
Appearance	is interest in oneself improving or worsening?
Attention span	is it improving or decreasing?

Sadness occurs in short bouts and may be realistically based on the impending loss of family, of independence or of life itself. It may have been triggered by planning a will or funeral, and saying 'goodbye'. Patients with sadness rather than depression are normally able to express and discuss their feelings in a rational and philosophical way.

℞ Remedy

Non-pharmacological management

Allow time to talk with the patient and encourage them to talk about the following:

- their fears about uncontrolled symptoms or the effects of drugs
- the process of dying and what happens after death

- any 'unfinished business' and what can be done to achieve important goals
- unsatisfied needs, wishes and worries
- real or imagined problems relating to dealings with the staff or other patients.

Talk to the members of the caring team and the family about the patient's worries and any sense of guilt felt by the patient.

Seek all available support (e.g. nurse, relatives, hospital chaplain, representatives from the same religion or country of origin as the patient) to discuss and deal with any cultural, social or religious issues that you may not be able to deal with yourself. Different cultures and faiths adopt different attitudes to suffering and illness and sharing of emotions. These need to be understood and dealt with appropriately, and serious offence can be taken as a result of making a mistake due to lack of understanding of cultural or religious practices or beliefs.

Remember that some people will simply not wish to talk. Homer expressed it like this:

> Eyes wet with tears, he spoke and her ladyship his mother heard him ...
> 'Child, why do you weep? What grief is this? Out with it, tell me, both of us should know.'
> Akhilleus, fast in battle as a lion, groaned and said 'Why tell you what you know?'[2]

Pharmacological management

Antidepressants need to be continued for a minimum of 3 weeks, but preferably for 6 weeks, in order to assess their effectiveness properly. Starting treatment within 6 weeks of death does not really allow time for benefit to be seen, so if depression is suspected, treatment needs to be started early on.

Tricyclic antidepressants

These drugs may take several weeks to become effective. Amitriptyline and dosulepin are more sedative than imipramine and lofepramine. All tricyclic antidepressants can cause difficulty with passing urine, a dry mouth and hypotension. Increasing the dose slowly will reduce the risk of these side-effects. The tricyclics interact with amiodarone and increase the risk of ventricular arrhythmias.

At lower doses, tricyclics can be used as co-analgesics. Any analgesic effect is probably independent of the antidepressant effects.

Selective serotonin reuptake inhibitors (SSRIs)

This group includes citalopram, fluoxetine and sertraline. They have fewer of the side-effects associated with the tricyclics, and are less sedating, but are also slower to act.

Some points about SSRIs are worth remembering.

- Headache, nausea and vomiting are among the side-effects.
- There is a risk of gastric bleeding in patients taking NSAIDs.
- There is an interaction with St John's Wort (hypericum) which patients can buy over the counter, so always ask patients about this and advise them to discontinue this herbal remedy.
- Fluoxetine increases blood levels of carbamazepine and phenytoin, with the risk of toxicity.

Having said this, the SSRIs are generally better tolerated by cancer patients. However, it should be noted that severe nocturnal agitation associated with confusion and hallucinations has occurred in patients with cerebral tumours who were treated with SSRIs.

St John's Wort

Many patients will choose to buy St John's Wort (hypericum) in the misguided belief that because it is 'natural' it is therefore harmless. There are two problems here. First, the drug is not regulated, so the amount and effectiveness of hypericum may vary from batch to batch and according to the manufacturer. Secondly, it interacts with several drugs by induction of cytochrome P_{450}, with the following possible outcomes.

Drug	*Interaction*
Anticonvulsants	Reduced blood levels: increased risk of seizures
Ciclosporin	Reduced blood levels: increased transplant rejection risk
Contraceptives (oral)	Reduced efficacy and risk of unintended pregnancy
Digoxin	Reduced blood levels
HIV protease inhibitors	Reduced blood levels: possible loss of HIV suppression
HIV non-nucleoside reverse transcriptase inhibitors	Reduced blood levels: possible loss of HIV suppression
SSRIs	Increased serotogenic effects
Theophylline	Reduced blood levels with loss of control of asthma
Triptans	Increased serotogenic effects
Warfarin	Reduced anticoagulation

E Extra information

Differentiation between sadness and depression is a matter of picking up cues and pointers, of allowing patients to express their fears and of offering them our sympathetic support.

Remember, too, that antidepressants are not intended to make patients 'happy'. The injudicious use of an antidepressant may cause unnecessary sedation, constipation and dry mouth, thus making the patient feel worse. There is substantial evidence that most depression in advanced cancer is caused by inadequate control of pain and other symptoms.

The biological indicators – disturbed sleep, constipation, loss of appetite, loss of weight and loss of libido – can all be direct effects of terminal illness. So too can weakness and emotional lability, with a tendency to cry more readily than usual.

Always bear in mind that the presence of organic disease may contribute to the patient's dysthymic state. Cerebral metastases or metabolic disturbances (e.g. hypercalcaemia) may result in a severe alteration in mood.

Depression can often be traced to concrete life circumstances. Try to:

- facilitate communication with family members
- help to minimise financial burdens
- diminish the impact of major changes in body image
- sensitise staff to the emotional needs of patients.

If appropriate, seek the help of a social worker or counsellor to help the patient and family members to cope with these issues.

References

1 Doyle D, Hanks GW, Cherny N *et al. The Oxford Textbook of Palliative Medicine.* Oxford: Oxford University Press; 2004.

2 Homer. *Iliad* 1: 357–65. Quoted in Galeazzi O. Truth, disease and prognosis. In: Surbone A, Zwitter M, editors. *Communication with the Cancer Patient.* New York: Annals of the New York Academy of Sciences, Vol. 809; 1997.

Further reading

- Geddes JR. Managing depressive disorder: how can the GP best help? *New Generalist.* 2004; **2:** 15–18.
- Geddes JR, Butler R, Hatcher S. Depressive disorders in adults. In: *Clinical Evidence.* London: BMJ Publishing Group; 2004. pp. 249–52.
- Laird B, Mitchell J. The assessment and management of depression in the terminally ill. *Eur J Palliat Care.* 2005; **12:** 101–4.
- Lloyd Williams M. Diagnosis and treatment of depression in palliative care. *Eur J Palliat Care.* 2002; **9:** 1860–8.
- Wernecke U *et al.* How effective is St John's Wort? The evidence revisited. J *Clin Psychiatry.* 2004; **66:** 611–17.

Chapter 28

Diarrhoea

> I have finally kum to the konklusion, that a good reliable sett ov bowels is wurth much more tu a man than enny quantity ov brains.
>
> Henry Wheeler Shaw (1818–1885), *Josh Billings: his sayings*

Introduction

In this text, diarrhoea refers to the passage of more than three unformed stools in 24 hours. It is important to check what the patient means when they refer to 'diarrhoea.'

Diarrhoea is less common than constipation among cancer patients.

C Consider

Is this true diarrhoea or spurious diarrhoea?

Spurious diarrhoea, due to faecal impaction, is mainly a profuse watery mucoid discharge. Some degree of faecal matter is always present in true diarrhoea. Steatorrhoea is characterised by offensive stools that are pale, fatty and difficult to flush away.

Is the patient on opioids? If so, are they actually suffering from constipation with overflow (spurious diarrhoea)?

Other causes of diarrhoea include the following:

- carcinoid tumours secreting hormones (rare)
- chemotherapy, particularly with fluorouracil, cisplatin and mitomycin
- colon or rectal tumours (due to partial obstruction or mucus secretion)
- certain drugs, including antibiotics, H_2-blockers, proton-pump inhibitors and SSRI antidepressants
- gastrectomy
- ileo-colic fistula
- infection
- ileum or jejunum resections
- laxatives in inappropriate doses
- malabsorption associated with cancer of the head of the pancreas
- radiotherapy to the abdomen or pelvis
- ulcerative colitis, Crohn's disease and steatorrhoea.

A Assess

Take a careful history from the patient, paying particular attention to the nature and consistency of the stools. Is there steatorrhoea or melaena?

Take a full drug history, giving particular attention to laxatives, antibiotics and antacids containing magnesium salts.

Carry out an abdominal examination, which may reveal a loaded colon.

A rectal examination is essential in order to detect faecal impaction and look for an empty but ballooned rectum, which indicates a higher faecal obstruction. Look for local colonic or rectal pathology which might cause diarrhoea.

Remember that diarrhoea could be caused by infection or biochemical upset, so check the corrected calcium concentration to exclude hypercalcaemia (which causes constipation).

If infection is considered to be a likely cause, perform stool culture. Most cases of infectious diarrhoea are viral and will resolve before the organism has been isolated. It is worth noting that diarrhoea due to either *Shigella* or *Clostridium difficile* may be exacerbated by opioids.

℞ Remedy

Explain the situation properly to the patient and carers.

Ensure that, where possible, the patient is involved in deciding on the use and dosage of any causative drugs, particularly laxatives.

The treatment depends on the cause. The common causes and treatments are briefly listed below.

Antibiotics

Bowel flora may be altered and diarrhoea will settle when the antibiotic course is completed, but exclude *Clostridium difficile*.

Carcinoid syndrome

Try octreotide or $5HT_3$ antagonists.

Faecal impaction

Enemas and suppositories should be used to clear the local blockage.

Ileal resection

Colestyramine should be used. It is interesting to note that colestyramine, when used to treat pruritus resulting from obstructive jaundice, can actually cause diarrhoea.

Intestinal disease (Crohn's or ulcerative colitis)

Sulfasalazine or steroids should be used.

Laxatives

Discontinue, review, and then restart at a more appropriate dose.

Malabsorption and steatorrhoea

Try pancreatic enzymes. Since gastric acids will destroy these, you should also give a proton pump inhibitor.

Non-specific

Try codeine 30–60 mg every 4–6 hours or loperamide 2–4 mg every 6 hours.

NSAIDs

Stopping or changing to another NSAID should be effective.

Radiotherapy induced

Ondansetron or colestyramine should be used.

Check that the patient's symptoms are resolving, and reassess the cause if they are not.

E Extra information

Laxatives, antibiotics and magnesium-containing antacids are drugs that are commonly used in patients with advanced cancer who are on opioids. All of these drugs can cause diarrhoea.

Opioid drugs are the mainstay of symptomatic management of diarrhoea. If the patient's cancer pain is controlled, and there is no other indication to increase the current dose of centrally acting opioids, loperamide should be added. Loperamide is a synthetic opioid derivative that, in therapeutic doses, is devoid of central effects. The maximum recommended daily dose is 16 mg, but this can be safely increased in cases of severe diarrhoea. In practice, the number of capsules that the patient can be expected to swallow may limit the dose that can be tolerated.

Further reading

No relevant journal papers were identified.

Chapter 29

Dysphagia

A good kitchen is a good apothecaries' shop.

William Bullein (d. 1576)

Introduction

Dysphagia, or difficulty in swallowing, occurs in around 10–12% of hospice patients.

To swallow effectively requires several normal functions:

- intact muscle and nerve function
- lip closure to prevent food leakage
- saliva for lubrication
- teeth to chew the food
- tongue mobility to push food to the pharynx.

Thus dysphagia can have various causes. The commonest is probably a dry mouth.

C Consider

Is the problem true dysphagia or pain on swallowing?

If it is true dysphagia, is it caused by a neurological deficit or by obstruction? Mechanical obstruction initially causes difficulty with solids only, whereas neuromuscular defects cause difficulty with solids and liquids.

Dysphagia may occur in neurological illness such as motor neuron disease, or may be the result of a benign stricture, but the main malignant causes are as follows:

- head and neck cancer
- mediastinal nodes compressing the oesophagus
- oesophageal cancer
- stomach cancer.

Oesophageal thrush should be considered, as it may be present even if oral thrush is absent.

Think about the implications of dysphagia, including weight loss and the associated effects of altered body image, on both the patient and the immediate family. Weight loss is a constant and visible reminder of disease progression.

A Assess

Is the difficulty due to discomfort or pain only, or does food stick in the throat?

Does the patient have difficulty swallowing solids, liquids or both?

Aspiration risk

There is always some risk of aspiration and this must be considered. Look out for the following:

- altered voice during eating (due to food on the vocal cords)

- cough on swallowing
- exhaustion when eating because it takes so long to swallow food
- pneumonia – is it aspiration pneumonia?
- wet sounds when eating (due to fluid in the airways).

℞ Remedy

Treat any cause of painful swallowing, such as sore mouth, a dry mouth or oral or oesophageal infection (e.g. candida).

Advise a soft or liquid diet and seek the advice of a dietitian.

General measures

Improving swallowing

- Eating cold food after throat surgery speeds the recovery of sensation.
- Varying the temperature and texture of foods aids recovery of the swallowing mechanisms.
- Chewing food for longer stimulates the swallowing reflex.
- If there is some loss of sensation in the mouth, encourage the patient to try to move food to an area where sensation is intact.
- Turn the head to the paralysed side to move food to the intact side of the throat.
- Fizzy drinks increase the sensation and awareness of a liquid bolus.
- Thickened or purėed food is easier to swallow when there is poor neuromuscular coordination.

Reducing the risk of aspiration

- Do not let the patient eat alone, but also do not distract them while they are eating.
- Encourage the patient to sit as upright as possible.
- Encourage them to swallow twice to stimulate oesophageal peristalsis.
- Thickened foods are easier to swallow.

Specific treatments

Dilatation

Dilating a malignant stricture using endoscopy takes a few minutes and can improve swallowing. About one-third of patients will need to have the procedure repeated.

Intubation

This procedure usually involves a general anaesthetic and may require the tube to be sutured in place via a laparotomy. The oesophagus is dilated prior to tube placement.

Nine out of ten patients benefit, but tubes can be associated with the following problems:

- blockage – advise the patient to take a fizzy drink with and after each meal to help clear food debris
- pain – the tube may have moved
- tumour regrowth and obstruction – laser treatment should re-canalise.

An oesophageal tube may become blocked with food, so to help to reduce this risk, food should be soft. Avoid stringy and pithy foods (e.g. oranges). Medications should be either crushed or given in a liquid formulation. Patients on sustained-release medications must have their medication reviewed and should be aware that they must not crush the tablets.

Laser

Laser debulking of tumour overgrowth in the lumen of the oesophagus helps about 90% of patients, but may need to be repeated every 6 weeks or so.

Nasogastric feeding

This is of value mainly if patients can swallow some food and fluids, and it is used for short-term nutritional support. Oesophageal ulceration can occur and the tube can be uncomfortable to pass and to retain.

Percutaneous endoscopic gastrostomy (PEG) tube feeding

PEG tube placement is simpler to perform than open gastrostomy. It is better tolerated than a nasogastric tube but cannot be performed if there is ascites present. Previous abdominal surgery or a gastric ulcer may render the procedure difficult or completely infeasible.

Radiotherapy

Intracavity or external beam radiotherapy may be used to reduce tumour size and improve swallowing. This treatment is not instantly effective, and this should be borne in mind.

Steroids

Dexamethasone at a dose of 8 mg daily can reduce peri-tumour oedema and thus improve swallowing in malignancies of the oesophagus. Dexamethasone can be given subcutaneously, or if necessary soluble prednisolone, 60 mg daily, could be given orally. The effect may not be seen for a few days.

Review the patient regularly to assess the success of the treatment employed.

E Extra information

Pain on swallowing can be caused by excess acid. Antacids or proton pump inhibitors should be tried. If thrush infection is suspected, treat with fluconazole or a similar systemic antifungal agent, but be aware of the possibility of interactions (e.g. antacids reduce the absorption of ketoconazole). Check for possible interactions with other prescribed medication.

Using a Doidy cup or a cutaway cup (*see* Figure 29.1) avoids the need to tilt the head while drinking. A polystyrene cup can be cut away using a sharp knife, or the occupational therapist may be able to supply a Doidy cup, which is also available from most retailers that specialise in the provision of aids for disabled people.

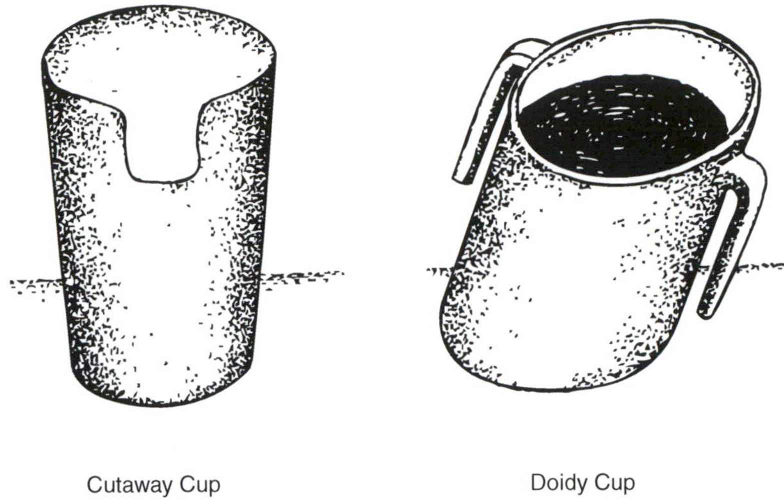

Figure 29.1 Cutaway cup and Doidy cup.

When it becomes difficult even to swallow saliva, the use of scopolamine patches every third day may reduce salivation and offer some symptomatic relief.

Development of a tracheo-oesophageal fistula is usually a pre-terminal event. Patients with this problem cough after eating, usually bringing up fluid which may include food that has been recently consumed. A small fistula may be sealed temporarily with an oesophageal tube, but the usual outcome is aspiration pneumonia. The decision as to whether or not to try to treat this event with antibiotics should be made on an individual basis.

Further reading

- Roe J. Oropharyngeal dysphagia in advanced non-head and neck malignancy. *Eur J Palliat Care.* 2005; **12:** 229–32.

Chapter 30

Fatigue

Life is one long process of getting tired.

Samuel Butler (1835–1902)

Introduction

Fatigue is almost universal among cancer sufferers, and patients use a variety of words to describe their energy levels. 'Tired', 'exhausted' or 'no energy' are common expressions. In this chapter, we shall use the word 'fatigue' to describe a range of symptoms from tiredness to inability to function normally due to lack of energy.

Several definitions exist, but the National Comprehensive Cancer Network (NCCN) definition of fatigue is 'a persistent subjective sense of tiredness, related to cancer or cancer treatment, that interferes with normal functioning'.[1]

Fatigued patients lose motivation, mental concentration and manual capacity to work.

All patients will report fatigue more often when undergoing radiotherapy or chemotherapy.

This subjective view is difficult to measure in terms of a patient's performance status, because some patients will 'push themselves to their limits' and assess the progress of their disease by monitoring their ability to keep going. Others will adopt a more leisurely lifestyle that does not make as many demands on their mental or physical energy at an earlier stage in their illness. Some patients can be objectively assessed more easily than others.[2]

Various instruments have been proposed for measuring fatigue, ranging from visual analogue scales, through numerical Likert-type scales to the 54-item Profile of Fatigue-Related Symptoms.[3]

Fatigue is difficult to manage, partly because patients vary so much in their presentation and their coping abilities.

Think about the similarity between fatigue and weakness, and make sure that you know exactly which the patient is describing.

C Consider

Is the weakness generalised or localised?

Think about the things that could be making the patient feel tired and generally weak:

- anaemia
- anorexia
- biochemical or metabolic upsets (e.g. diabetes, hypothyroidism)
- cachexia
- chemotherapy
- depression and anxiety
- hypotension
- infection

- pain
- radiotherapy
- sleep deprivation.

Localised weaknesses may be due to the following:

- brain metastases
- cord compression (affects both legs)
- cerebrovascular accident (CVA) (onset will be sudden, not gradual)
- nerve damage (may be associated with pain).

A Assess

Take a history from the patient, bearing the possible causes in mind. Conduct a basic examination, including blood pressure, which falls as the patient loses weight. Antihypertensive drug doses may need to be reviewed.

If there is pre-existing metabolic disease, check the degree of control from recent blood tests and repeat these to assess current disease status and control.

A full blood count will reveal any underlying anaemia. Because fatigue usually has a multi-factorial aetiology, correction of slowly progressive anaemia in patients with advanced cancer may not overcome the feeling of fatigue.

If weakness is localised, conduct appropriate tests to determine the cause.

℞ Remedy

Fatigue is so variable that it is essential to have an individual management plan for each patient. However, there are a few areas that are common to all patients.

General measures

Every patient needs support and some counselling to help them to cope with the effects of advancing illness.

Suggest to all patients that they conserve energy and pace themselves, by delegating tasks and making adequate time for rest and relaxation. Encourage the patient to keep as active as possible and to set realistic, achievable goals. Practical support (e.g. a home help to undertake certain tasks in order to allow the patient to conserve energy) should be provided as appropriate.

All fatigued patients should be assessed by the occupational therapist to discuss their activities of daily living and think about any modifications to the home which may be required to help them to continue to live a relatively normal life for as long as possible.

The physiotherapist can help the patient to make the best use of their energy and can also help them to retain their mobility.

Specific measures

Anaemia

Fatigued patients who are anaemic may respond to weekly erythropoietin. How this works is uncertain. It may be due to correction of the anaemia, or there may be a direct effect on the erythropoietin receptors in the brain and other tissues.

Biochemical and metabolic disorders

Correct biochemical upsets, including:

- hypercalcaemia
- hypokalaemia (which may be due to diuretics or steroids).

Correct metabolic disturbances, including:

- blood sugar
- thyroid dysfunction.

Depression

Is the patient depressed? This could either be causing, or could be caused by, the fatigue. Depression may present as chronic fatigue in the absence of any history of sleeplessness. Treat any underlying depression with an antidepressant such as amitriptyline, dosulepin or lofepramine. Depression may present with anxiety that prevents the patient from getting to sleep, or as early-morning wakening. Sleep improvement should be seen after a few days, but an antidepressant effect may take 2 to 6 weeks.

Nutrition

Check that the patient is eating and drinking well enough. Reinforce the fact that eating what they want, when they feel like it, is more valuable than rigid meal-times.

Pain

Make sure that pain is well controlled.

Sleep

Attend to any physical discomfort that is preventing sleep. Check that steroids are not being taken late in the afternoon or in the early evening. Only prescribe hypnotics if they are required. There is no place for the routine prescribing of night sedation. Instead, it should be prescribed on an individual basis after assessment of need.

E Extra information

Radiotherapy and chemotherapy commonly cause fatigue. The mechanism is not fully understood, but it is thought to be related to an increase in basal metabolic rate, together with the metabolic effects of tumour breakdown, in addition to the obvious psychological and emotional reactions to treatment.

Prednisolone (10–30 mg) or dexamethasone (4 mg in a single morning dose) may help radiotherapy patients who are suffering from fatigue.

The patient's fatigue can often be a source of major stress in close relationships. Adequate time should be allowed for the patient to express their feelings and anxieties. Occasionally, an anxiolytic such as diazepam may be required.

A paper published in the journal *Annals of Oncology* reports that fatigue may not be related to renal, thyroid, hepatic or haematological function,[4] but that many fatigued patients had high depression scores.

References

1 Mock V, Atkinson A, Barserick A *et al.* NCCN practice guidelines for cancer-related fatigue. *Oncology.* 2000; **14:** 151–61.
2 Piper BF. Measuring fatigue. In: Frank-Stromberg M, Olsen SJ, editors. *Instruments for Clinical Health-Care Research.* Sudbury, MA: Jones and Bartlett; 1997. pp. 486–7.
3 Piper BF. Important measures of fatigue. In: Frank-Stromberg M, Olsen SJ, editors. *Instruments for Clinical Health-Care Research.* Sudbury, MA: Jones and Bartlett; 1997. pp. 494–6.
4 Dimeo F, Schmittel A, Fietz T *et al.* Physical performance, depression, immune status and fatigue in patients with hematological malignancies after treatment. *Ann Oncol.* 2004; **15:** 1237–42.

Further reading

- Brown H. The management of cancer-related fatigue. *Eur J Palliat Care.* 2004; **11:** 16–18.
- Lane I. Managing cancer-related fatigue in palliative care. *Nurs Times.* 2005; **101:** 38–41.
- Pedersen L, Munch TN, Groenvold M. The treatment of fatigue in palliative care patients. *Eur J Palliat Care.* 2003; **10:** 225–9.
- Sharpe M, Wilks D. Fatigue (ABC of psychological medicine series). *BMJ.* 2002; **325:** 480–83.
- Summers E. Understanding the nature of cancer-related fatigue. *Nurs Times.* 2005; **101:** 30–32.
- Tonks NF, Dean A. The causes of cancer-related fatigue and approaches to its management. *Prof Nurse.* 2004; **19:** 503–7.

Chapter 31

Fistulae

> A bad state of health is often joined with a fistula in ano, and the mischief, after the cure of the ulcer, has many times fallen upon other parts, and particularly the lungs, and has brought on asthmas, spittings of blood, and consumptions.
>
> William Heberden (1710–1801)[1]

Introduction

A fistula is an abnormal connection between two hollow organs, or between a hollow organ and the surface of the body.

Fistulae may form as a result of the malignancy itself eating into the tissues, after infection or following surgery or radiotherapy.

Once it has formed, a fistula often fails to heal for the following reasons.

- The exudate keeps the surfaces wet and prevents healing from taking place.
- There is often infection present.
- There is often a deep-seated necrotic tumour mass underlying the fistula.

Necrotic tumour is usually not treatable as such, but check whether an abscess is underlying, as this should be drained and treated with antibiotics.

C Consider

Why has this fistula formed? Is it due to the cancer, surgery, radiotherapy or infection?

How are the patient and the family or lay carers coping with the fistula?

What treatment has the patient received? Is more treatment required or is it feasible?

Is there odour present, suggesting infection?

A Assess

Check where the fistula has formed, how long it has been present and how it is affecting the patient. Does the patient understand how and why it has formed?

These lesions are usually a source of great distress to patients. Ask about pain and the appearance and smell.

Is the fistula resulting in isolation as a result of the effects on body image or the feelings of embarrassment about the associated odour or any leakage of exudate?

Is infection present? Fungating wounds are often painful and smelly, but some patients have kept them hidden for a long time.

What does the patient think can be done? Are their expectations realistic and are they being met as far as possible?

℞ Remedy

Every fistula requires individual management.

General measures

Pain and smell due to infection should be treated with analgesia and antibiotics. Metronidazole gel is soothing and helps to control malodour.

Barrier creams may help to reduce the soreness of the surrounding skin.

A colostomy bag placed over the fistula will help to collect excessive discharge.

Specific sites

Buccal fistula

The constant leakage of saliva and food can have adverse effects on the patient's well-being.

A plug of gauze may seal off a small fistula.

A Silastic foam plug made from a cast of the fistula and retained by a simple dressing may reduce fluid loss in larger fistulae. Making two plugs allows one to be used while the other is washed.

Transdermal or sublingual hyoscine may help to reduce the volume of saliva produced, or a tricyclic antidepressant may help to overcome depression and also reduce salivation as a beneficial side-effect.

External intestinal fistula

A colostomy bag fitted over the opening may help to collect effluent when a fistula develops between the bowel and the abdominal wall. Extra-large appliances may be required to cover more than one fistula. The advice of a stoma nurse on skin protection and on the selection of the best type of bag is invaluable.

Octreotide administered by subcutaneous injection or syringe driver may help to reduce the volume of secretions from the fistula.

Recto-vaginal, recto-vesical or vesico-vaginal fistulae

Surgery should be considered if the patient is fit enough and has a suitable prognosis. A colostomy and/or urinary diversion can bring complete symptomatic relief.

Reducing the dose of laxatives or giving low doses of loperamide or codeine phosphate (if the patient is not taking opioids) will allow the stool to become firmer.

Vaginal tampons may also help. Use a tampon that expands horizontally rather than vertically (e.g. 'Lil-lets' rather than 'Tampax').

Tracheo-oesophageal fistula

Development of a tracheo-oesophageal fistula is usually a pre-terminal event. Patients with this problem cough after eating, usually bringing up fluid which may be recognisable as what has been recently consumed. A small fistula may be sealed temporarily with an oesophageal tube, but the usual outcome is aspiration pneumonia. The decision as to whether or not to try to treat this event with antibiotics should be made on an individual basis.

E Extra information

Many fistulae are not 'treatable', so the aim becomes one of keeping the lesion as odourless and comfortable as possible, while trying to enable the patient to continue to live as normal a life as possible.

Sometimes radiotherapy or cryotherapy may be of value, but these need to be discussed with a specialist. Large exophytic masses or lesions on the surface, with no direct continuation to a deeper tumour, are the most amenable to treatment.

Review the patient regularly and provide emotional support while evaluating the management.

Seek the advice of the specialist wound management team.

Be realistic about the outcomes of any interventions, and do not give the patient false hope that an effective treatment is available.

Reference

1 Heberden W. *Commentaries on the History and Cure of Diseases.* London: T. Payne and Son; 1802.

Further reading

No relevant journal papers were identified.

Chapter 32

Fungating wounds

> A wound should be bound with clean white bandages, else there be harmful effects. He should wash his hands before treating anyone.
>
> Heinrich von Pfolspeundt, fifteenth-century German war surgeon, *Buch der Bundth-Erntznei*

Introduction

The presence of a wound that refuses to heal is something that patients simply cannot ignore. The discharge, bleeding, pain and the need to have regular dressings all act as reminders of the advancing disease. About 10% of all cancer patients will develop skin secondaries, with an average survival of 3 months after this development.

Skin lesions are of two basic types:

- localised skin involvement (e.g. a fungating breast skin lesion)
- generalised skin metastases – these are a sign of very late disease.

Local invasion of tumour into the tissues results in small emboli in the lymphatics and blood vessels, which threaten the tissue viability. A cascade of events follows, consisting of infarction, necrosis and infection, often with anaerobes. Most local skin lesions are associated with breast cancer and lung cancer, and the usual sites where they occur are either on the chest wall or on the scalp.

C Consider

The aim of treatment needs to be realistically thought through. Is one looking for cure and complete healing, or is the focus on palliation? Often it is the latter, in which case one should then think about the following:

- bleeding
- discharge
- infection
- pain
- psychological effects on the patient and their family
- smell.

Has the patient already had chemotherapy, radiotherapy or surgery (e.g. a toilet mastectomy)?

Has palliative radiotherapy been considered? It can cause dramatic shrinkage and occasionally healing of a tumour.

Palliative chemotherapy for a fungating breast carcinoma may result in regression of the skin lesion.

Superficial palliative radiotherapy may be offered to delay tumour growth when the skin is still intact. After fungation has occurred, the situation is more difficult to manage, but superficial radiotherapy may be of value in reducing tumour bulk and arresting haemorrhage. This may allow healing to commence, but many patients will not live long enough to see complete healing.

Seek the advice of the specialist wound-management team.

A Assess

The management of these lesions needs to be planned individually and depends partly on where the patient is being cared for and how frequently the wound needs attention.

Assess the need to attend to the following:

- bleeding
- comfort of dressings and the wound generally
- coping and psychological issues
- cosmetic appearance
- exudate
- infection
- lifestyle and ability to continue social contact
- odour
- pain.

℞ Remedy

Bleeding

Apply gauze soaked in adrenaline 1:1000 or sucralfate liquid to the bleeding points, or use calcium alginate dressings. Saline spray or saline soaks may facilitate removal of dressings with minimal discomfort and risk of trauma causing further bleeding.

Consider superficial radiotherapy to control persistent bleeding.

Comfort of dressings and the wound generally

This is a very individual choice and may require a period of 'trial and error.' If dressings are being prescribed by the GP, and several new ones are tried, think about the cost of each prescription and discuss the option of pre-payment if the patient is not exempt from paying for prescriptions and it is thought that this might cost less. It might not be a realistic option for patients with a short prognosis.

Coping and psychological issues

Every patient with a fungating wound will be anxious about leakage, odour and their appearance, either because of a bulky dressing or because of a visible lesion (e.g. on the scalp). Sensitivity and support are vital, and odour-controlling and leak-proof dressings along with explanation, reassurance and understanding will all help.

Cosmetic appearance

Keeping bulk to a minimum and trying to preserve as normal an appearance as possible should be the aim. It may be easier to make a dressing look reasonably normal under clothing, but scalp wounds are more difficult to hide.

Exudate

High-absorbency dressings with leak-proof seals should be used if possible. Additional padding on top 'just in case' will give extra reassurance but also adds some bulk. Protect the surrounding skin with a barrier cream.

Infection

Local infection is almost unavoidable as a warm, moist, protein-rich exudate provides perfect culture conditions for bacteria. Antibiotics should ideally be prescribed according to the results of swabs taken for culture and sensitivity, but if it is necessary to prescribe before these results are available, flucloxacillin or, for those allergic to penicillin, erythromycin or trimethoprim are reasonable choices. Metronidazole is needed for anaerobes, and metronidazole gel is useful for the associated odour.

Staphylococcus aureus is among the commonest organisms, but the possibility of MRSA must be remembered.

Cephalosporins are excellent, but they are associated with an increased risk of diarrhoea due to *Clostridium difficile*.

Lifestyle and ability to continue social contact

The type of dressing that is needed may depend on the patient's lifestyle. Patients should be encouraged to continue to attend social events and be made aware that a less-bulky dressing may be possible for the short period during which they are out in company. These patients should also be encouraged to keep looking after themselves, using make-up, having their hair styled or doing whatever makes them feel good about themselves for as long as they can do so and wish to make the effort.

Odour

Good ventilation is essential in order to minimise lingering aromas. Deodorisers on top of the dressing may help. However, replacing one smell with another one from an 'air freshener' fools no one!

Metronidazole gel or oral metronidazole for a deeper infection should help. One possibility is that, as anaerobes are eradicated, aerobic bacteria may increase in number and cause infection. Regular swabs for culture and sensitivity will confirm this, but a short break in the use of metronidazole every 7 days or so often allows the bacterial colonies to stabilise.

Charcoal dressings and dressings that seal the edges of wounds are also helpful.

Pain

Pain may be due to any of the following:

- dressings sticking
- infection
- nerve damage.

Treat infections, use non-stick dressings and offer analgesia a short time before dressing changes if the pain is associated with this procedure. Suitable analgesics include the following:

- oral morphine (immediate release)
- subcutaneous diamorphine
- inhaled 'Entonox' (nitrous oxide/oxygen)
- NSAIDs.

Aluminium hydroxide/magnesium hydroxide suspension ('Maalox') applied topically may relieve burning sensations.

Natural yogurt applied topically is also reported to be helpful.

E Extra information

Management goals should be realistic. Review them regularly and assess them with regard to alteration in lesion size, colour, odour, pain, etc.

It is important to remember that the quality of the patient's life must be preserved at all times. Consider the impact of this type of lesion on the patient's self-esteem and how intimacy between the patient and their partner may be affected. The patient may be reluctant to discuss this issue or to initiate such a discussion, but it should not be overlooked.

Do not assume that a man is aware of the extent of his partner's breast lesion. One of the authors attended a woman with breast cancer, and it was only on visiting the couple's home that it became obvious that they lived under the same roof, but did not share a bedroom, and the husband knew nothing of the fungating wound that his wife had concealed for several months.

Further reading

- Bird C. Managing malignant fungating wounds. *Prof Nurse.* 2000; **15:** 253–6.
- Kelly N. Malodorous fungating wounds: a review of the current literature. *Prof Nurse.* 2002; **17:** 323–6.
- Naylor W. Palliative management of fungating wounds. *Eur J Palliat Care.* 2003; **10:** 93–7.

Chapter 33

Halitosis

> Miss Debary, Susan and Sally made their appearance, and I was as civil to them as their bad breath would allow me.
>
> Jane Austen (1775–1815)[1]

Introduction

Halitosis, or foul-smelling breath, has been recognised and treated in various ways for centuries. Thousands of years ago, Jewish women used a peppercorn carried in their mouths as a breath freshener.[2]

Queen Elizabeth I 'carried at her belt a small bag filled with sweets'. She sucked them to disguise her fetid breath, associated with her decayed teeth, probably not recognising that they were making the problem worse.[2]

Halitosis can be a serious problem in the care of a terminally ill patient, creating a barrier between the patient and their family and causing social isolation.

C Consider

Halitosis can have several causes, which can arise from oral, respiratory tract or gut problems. And don't forget the simple things like spicy food or garlic!

Oral causes include:

- bleeding from an infection or tumour in the mouth
- infection (e.g. anaerobes, or occasionally candida or herpes)
- necrotic tumour of the oral cavity
- poor mouth hygiene with or without a dry mouth and periodontal disease.

Respiratory causes include:

- necrotic tumours anywhere in the respiratory tract
- sinus infection.

Gastrointestinal causes include:

- gastric stasis, often associated with a linitis plastica gastric cancer
- obstruction with faecal vomiting.

Other causes include:

- kidney failure
- liver failure.

A Assess

The nature of the smell of the breath may provide a clue to the cause.

Type of odour	*Possible cause*
'Sewer-like'	Anaerobic infection, look for: • intestinal obstruction • lung abscess or bronchiectasis • necrotic tumour of mouth or throat
Sweet/sickly	Pseudomonas pneumonia
Fishy or urine-like	Kidney failure
Musty or ammonia-like	Liver failure

℞ Remedy

General measures

- Avoid foods that may be responsible, such as garlic or spices.
- Maintain excellent oral hygiene, including denture cleaning and disinfection.
- Maintain a good fluid intake if possible, but think carefully before suggesting starting intravenous fluids if the prognosis is short.

Specific measures

Gastric stasis

Gastric stasis with reflux of stomach contents into the oesophagus may cause halitosis. This can be treated with drugs such as metoclopramide (10 mg four times daily) or domperidone (10–20 mg four times daily).

Mouth and oropharynx

Anaerobic infection of the gums often causes halitosis. It is easily treated with oral metronidazole (400 mg twice daily).

Bleeding in the mouth can be controlled with tranexamic acid 500 mg three times daily or applied locally.

Dentures must be cleaned regularly, preferably in 0.2% chlorhexidine gluconate (but not soaked in this solution). Good oral hygiene is essential.

A dry mouth should be treated with artificial saliva, and a reasonable fluid intake should be maintained.

Necrotic tumours of the oropharynx should be treated with topical or oral metronidazole, and 1% hydrogen peroxide mouthwashes should be given four times a day.

Lung

Anaerobic infection of the lungs can cause particularly troublesome halitosis. It may be treated with systemic metronidazole 250 mg three times daily, with the possible addition of amoxicillin 250–500 mg three times daily while the results of sputum culture are awaited.

E Extra information

If no obvious cause of halitosis can be found, it is reasonable to try a 5-day course of oral metronidazole, 200 mg three times a day.

References

1 Austen J. Extract from letter 27 (dated 20 November 1800). In: Le Faye D, editor. *Jane Austen's Letters.* Oxford: Oxford University Press; 1995.

2 Ring ME. *Dentistry: an illustrated history.* New York: Harry N Abrams; 1985.

Further reading

- Porter SR, Scully C. Oral malodour (halitosis). *BMJ.* 2006; **333:** 632–5.

Chapter 34

Hiccup

> Sneezing coming on, in the case of a person afflicted with hiccup, removes the hiccup.
>
> Hippocrates (460–357 BC), *Aphorisms* VI.13

Introduction

Hiccups are caused by spasms of the diaphragm leading to a sudden intake of breath, which is cut off when the vocal cords close quickly, causing the characteristic sound which gives rise to their onomatopoeic name.

Hiccups serve no known function, have no single reliable treatment and can be very exhausting for the patient, especially as they can persist for several days.

C Consider

Diaphragmatic spasm due to diaphragmatic irritation results in hiccups. The diaphragmatic irritation is often caused by gastric distension or liver enlargement, the diaphragmatic irritation being stimulated by involvement of two main nerve pathways, namely the vagus nerve and the phrenic nerve. Drugs and systemic causes must also be considered.

Drugs

- Barbiturates.
- Benzodiazepines.
- Steroids.

Stimulation of the phrenic nerve

- Brain tumours, especially brainstem.
- Diaphragmatic tumour invasion.
- Mediastinal tumour.
- Meningeal infiltration by tumour deposits.

Stimulation of the vagus nerve

- Abdominal distension (e.g. ascites).
- Distended stomach.
- Gastro-oesophageal reflux.
- Liver tumours.

Systemic causes

- Addison's disease.
- Hyponatraemia.
- Kidney failure.

A Assess

How long has the patient been hiccupping?

Did the hiccup start following any recent change in medication?

Do the hiccups stop at night? Psychogenic hiccups stop during sleep. Has there been any new psychological problem?

Has the patient had a stroke?

Has there been a recent irritation of the vagus nerve (e.g. tumours of neck, mediastinum, oesophagus and lung, or recent chest surgery)?

Carry out a general examination, looking for:

- CNS disturbance or pressure on the vagus nerve from tumour
- gastric distension
- signs of sepsis.

Check for:

- hypocalcaemia
- hyponatraemia
- uraemia.

℞ Remedy

Treatment of hiccup can be unsuccessful, and no single treatment can be guaranteed.

Stop any drugs that could be responsible (e.g. steroids).

Non-pharmacological treatments

These may give temporary relief and can be tried quite safely.

Pharyngeal stimulation

- Breath-holding or rebreathing into a paper bag. As the PCO_2 rises, hiccup should decrease, but it may restart after resuming normal breathing.
- Dry granulated sugar to eat.
- Iced water to sip, or crushed ice to eat.
- Lemon slices to suck.
- Massaging the soft palate or lifting the uvula with a cotton-bud.

Stimulation of the C5 dermatome

- Cold item behind the collar.
- Coolant spray to the back of the neck over the C5 dermatome.
- Massaging the back of the neck.

How these remedies work is unclear, but they probably interrupt the hiccup reflex arc.

Pharmacological treatments

Gastric distension

- Domperidone 10–20 mg four times daily *or*
- Metoclopramide 10 mg four times daily.

Both of these drugs are pro-kinetics and may promote gastric emptying. In addition, offer smaller but more frequent meals. Offer a defoaming antiflatulant such as simeticone to prevent distension due to gas.

Smooth muscle relaxation

- Baclofen 5 mg three times daily *or*
- Nifedipine 5 mg as required or three times daily.

Suppression of the hiccup reflex

- Chlorpromazine 25 mg. *Note:* This may cause drowsiness and hypotension and should only be used when symptoms are severe and intractable or other measures have failed.

Suppression of intracranial tumour CNS irritation

- Dexamethasone, starting with 16 mg daily *or*
- Phenytoin 200–300 mg at night.

Steroids can *cause* hiccups, so be aware of this when considering this treatment option.

E Extra information

Intractable hiccup can be very difficult to treat. Occasionally you may need to seek advice about two infrequently used treatments, namely:

- phrenic nerve block
- radiotherapy to mediastinal nodes.

Further reading

- Hardy J. The treatment of hiccups in terminal patients. *Eur J Palliat Care.* 2003; **10:** 192–3.

Chapter 35

Hypercalcaemia

To avoid delay, please have all your symptoms ready.
Anonymous (seen on a notice in a waiting room)

Introduction

Hypercalcaemia is defined as a corrected serum calcium concentration above 2.6 mmol/litre. Levels above 4.0 mmol/litre will cause death in a few days. Hypercalcaemia is treatable but may be missed, as the symptoms can be mild and the problem may remain undetected until the serum calcium level has risen to 3.0 mmol/litre or more.

It is essential to think about the possibility of hypercalcaemia in all patients with advanced cancer, and especially in those with lung and breast cancer, as these two malignancies account for half of all cases. Myeloma is not as commonly associated with the condition, but one-third of myeloma patients will develop hypercalcaemia.

C Consider

The cancers most commonly associated with hypercalcaemia are breast, bronchus (squamous-cell carcinoma), myeloma, lymphoma and leukaemia. Squamous-cell cancers of the head and neck and oesophagus, and genito-urinary cancers can all be associated with hypercalcaemia.

Symptoms of hypercalcaemia include the following:

- confusion
- constipation
- drowsiness, progressing to coma
- muscle weakness
- nausea and vomiting
- polyuria
- thirst
- tiredness.

If drowsiness, nausea, vomiting and thirst are present, suspect hypercalcaemia as the likely cause.

Most patients with hypercalcaemia have widespread disease and have a prognosis of several months, with an average of 3 to 4 months.

Bone metastases do not have to be present for hypercalcaemia to develop. About 20% of patients with hypercalcaemia will not have bone secondaries.

A Assess

Ask about the following:

- constipation
- muscle weakness

- nausea and vomiting
- polyuria
- thirst
- tiredness.

Assess the following:

- confusion
- dehydration, a major feature of hypercalcaemia due to polyuria and vomiting
- drowsiness.

Check the following:
- corrected serum calcium concentration (corrected for serum albumin, as ionised calcium represents about 50% of serum calcium)
- urea and electrolytes:
  - alkaline phosphatase is usually elevated (but is normal in myeloma)
  - blood urea, nitrogen and creatinine may be raised due to renal damage
  - chloride may be elevated in primary hyperparathyroidism
- ECG – bradycardia may be present, and ECG changes include a prolonged P–R interval, a reduced Q–T interval and wide T-waves.

℞ Remedy

The most important thing to remember is to rehydrate the patient with 2–3 litres of intravenous fluids per 24 hours.

Each day also check the following:

- corrected calcium levels
- urea and electrolytes in order to detect hypokalaemia and hyponatraemia.

Rehydration alone will seldom be sufficient to correct serum calcium levels, and drugs are usually required.

The drugs fall into four categories:

- bisphosphonates
- calcitonin
- plicamycin
- steroids.

Relevant pathophysiology of hypercalcaemia

Hypercalcaemia is caused by secretion of a tumour peptide called parathormone-releasing protein. This causes the release of calcium from bone via increased osteoclastic activity, and also a reduction in calcium excretion in the urine.

Bisphosphonates

Bisphosphonates inhibit osteoclast activity, thus correcting the hypercalcaemia, but may take 48 hours to become effective. About 20% of patients will not respond to bisphosphonates.

Bisphosphonates are given initially by infusion, followed by oral maintenance therapy. The following drugs are used:

- clodronate 1.5 g given over 4 hours
- disodium pamidronate 30–90 mg given over 2–4 hours
- ibandronic acid 2–4 mg given over 1–2 hours
- zoledronic acid 4 mg given over 15 minutes.

Zoledronic acid works faster and lasts for longer than the other drugs, but is more expensive.

Calcitonin

Calcitonin inhibits bone resorption by osteoclasts and encourages the excretion of calcium. It acts within a few hours and works for about one-third of patients.

Plicamycin

Plicamycin (formerly called mithromycin) is a cytotoxic antibiotic that blocks RNA synthesis and is toxic to osteoclasts. The dose is 25 mg/kg body weight over 2 hours, and about 80% of patients will show a fall in serum calcium levels over the next 72 hours. Plicamycin is toxic to the liver and kidneys and has been superseded by other drugs.

Steroids

Steroids have an inhibitory effect on osteoclasts in the laboratory, but are less effective in clinical practice. Their main use is in haematological malignancies, where prednisolone, 40–100 mg daily, is often effective.

E Extra information

Hypercalcaemia may occasionally be due to non-malignant causes. These include the following:

- primary hyperparathyroidism due to benign parathyroid adenomas. Treatment is by excision
- tamoxifen-induced flare reactions after starting on tamoxifen therapy
- vitamin D intoxication. Avoid preparations containing calcium and vitamins A and D.

Ranitidine and cimetidine increase renal blood flow and should be avoided.

Thiazide diuretics can exacerbate hypercalcaemia.

Further reading

- Anon. Osteonecrosis of the jaw with bisphosphonates. *Curr Probl Pharmacovigilance.* 2006; **31:** 4.
- Howell A. Tumour-induced hypercalcaemia. *Eur J Palliat Care.* 2002; **9:** 5–7.

Chapter 36

Itch

It is easy to stand a pain, but difficult to stand an itch.
Chang Ch'ao (Chinese sage) *Sweet Dream Shadows* (*c.* 1676)

Introduction

Itch occurs in about 10% of cancer patients. Itch and pain share the same nerve pathways, and itch is mediated via the opioid-receptor sites, which is why naloxone reduces itch.

A variety of itch mediators may be responsible, including bile salts, histamine, proteases and trypsin.

Being warm, dry, anxious or bored increases the awareness of itch.

C Consider

Local skin problems are the commonest cause of itch, and include the following:

- dermatitis
- dry skin (especially in the elderly)
- infections and infestations (fleas, mites, scabies)
- wet skin.

Drugs can cause itch for a variety of reasons, which are listed below.

Allergy

- Allopurinol.
- Carbamazepine.
- Nitrofurantoin.
- Penicillin.
- Streptomycin.
- Sulphonamides.

Histamine release

- Aspirin.
- Opioids (e.g. codeine and morphine; this is not dose related).
- X-ray contrast agents.

Liver cholestatis

- Captopril.
- Chlorpromazine.
- Steroids.
- Trimethoprim.

Itch may also be a result of the illness itself:

- Hodgkin's disease or non-Hodgkin's lymphoma ('type B symptoms')

- liver and biliary tree obstructive disease (the severity of the itch is not related to bilirubin level)
- paraneoplastic itch (an uncommon but important cause of generalised itching)
- renal failure
- skin infiltration by the malignancy.

A Assess

Ask when the itch started and whether there is any time relationship to starting a new medication.

Ask about new soaps and cosmetics.

Ask about the timing and severity of the itch. Does it waken the patient? If so, this suggests a systemic cause.

Examine the skin, looking for the following:

- excoriations in web spaces (scabies)
- inflammatory papules
- jaundice
- the 'butterfly' sign on the upper back (hepatobiliary disease).

On general examination, look for hepatomegaly and lymphadenopathy.

Blood tests

- Full blood count with differential white cell count.
- Liver function tests.
- Thyroxine and thyroid-stimulating hormone (TSH) (hyperthyroidism can cause itch).
- Urea and electrolytes.

℞ Remedy

General advice

Intact skin

- Use aqueous cream or emulsifying ointment as a soap substitute.
- Avoid hot baths.
- Wear cool, loose-fitting, cotton clothes.
- Dry skin by patting, not rubbing.
- Apply moisturiser to the skin.
- Sodium bicarbonate added to a cool bath can be very soothing.

Broken or macerated skin

- Avoid all powders.
- Use a hairdryer on a cool setting to dry the skin.
- For inflamed skin, use hydrocortisone cream for a few days.
- Ensure protection from excessive moisture.
- Yeast infections should be treated with antifungal creams.

Specific situations

Cholestasis

The usual cause is blockage of the common bile duct (CBD) by a tumour of the head of the pancreas. Stenting the CBD relieves both the jaundice and itch. Dexamethasone may help. Ondansetron 8 mg IV initially, followed by 8 mg twice daily orally, may help.

Colestyramine 4 g twice daily (if the patient can tolerate the taste) and steroids have been used with variable degrees of success in the treatment of itching associated with obstructive jaundice. Colestyramine is contraindicated in complete biliary obstruction.

Lymphoma

Cimetidine may be of value. The mechanism is unclear, but may be due to an inhibitory action on the liver enzymes.

Opioid-induced itch

Ondansetron 8 mg IV initially, followed by 8 mg twice daily orally may help. Opioid antagonists will stop the itch but will also stop the opioid easing the pain.

Paraneoplastic syndrome

Paroxetine may help by its action on the $5HT_3$ receptors, but may also cause sedation and nausea, which limits its usefulness.

Rashes and bites

Oily calamine or menthol (1–2%) in aqueous cream may be useful. Crotamiton cream may give relief.

Renal failure

Itch in renal failure probably has multiple causes. Around 70% of patients have localised itch which may respond to capsaicin cream. Generalised itch may respond to ondansetron 8 mg twice daily. Treat the renal failure as far as possible.

Skin infiltration by breast cancer

Try aspirin or another COX-1 NSAID. Think about the risk of gastric erosion.

E Extra information

Antihistamines are the usual symptomatic treatment for itching. Non-sedating antihistamines are only effective when the itch is associated with histamine wealing (e.g. dermatographism and urticaria). In all other conditions, sedative antihistamines are required.

Non-pharmaceutical approaches may help. For example, cucumber applied topically cools the skin and reduces itch.

Further reading

- Thorns A, Edmonds P. The management of pruritus in palliative care patients. *Eur J Palliat Care.* 2000; **7:** 9–12.
- Tomson N, Burrows N. Pruritus: causes and management. *Geriatr Med.* 2006; **35:** 35–41. (This paper looks at non-malignant and cancer-related causes of itch.)

Chapter 37

Jaundice

> A violent itching of the skin, without any eruption, is familiar to the jaundice and adds sometimes to the discomforts of old age.
>
> William Heberden (English physician, 1710–1801), *Commentaries on the History and Cures of Diseases*

Introduction

'Jaundice' is a descriptive term derived from an old French word meaning 'yellow coloured', and is not a diagnosis as such.

Jaundice causes yellowing of the skin and the whites of the eyes. The patient's urine becomes dark and their bowel motions become pale.

The presence of jaundice in a palliative care setting usually indicates that death is very near. Cancer infiltrating the liver sufficient to cause jaundice is associated with an average prognosis of 1 month at the most. The cause of the jaundice must be determined so that appropriate management can be offered to the patient.

The classification – determining whether the jaundice is of pre-hepatic, hepatic or post-hepatic origin – is probably of little relevance if the patient has a short prognosis.

C Consider

Think about the possible causes of jaundice, remembering that there are benign causes as well as those related to cancer:

- gallstones
- Gilbert's disease
- hepatitis A, B or C
- hepatotoxic drugs (e.g. alcohol, chlorpromazine, halothane)
- pancreatitis
- primary cancer of the ampulla of Vater, pancreas or cholangiocarcinoma
- secondary tumour infiltration of the liver.

A Assess

Is the jaundice painful?

Has the patient suffered from some other disease that could be causing the jaundice?

Assess the possibility that the jaundice could have an infectious basis.

Perform a general examination, check the size of the liver and look for tenderness.

Check for anaemia and exclude Gilbert's disease (familial non-haemolytic jaundice).

Perform liver function tests to assist in diagnosis and guide management.

Do not put the patient through the trauma of CT scanning, ultrasound scanning, cholangiography or liver biopsy unless it is likely that these will be used for a worthwhile management programme in a relatively fit patient.

℞ Remedy

Pain may indicate rapid stretching of the liver capsule. If this is suspected, treat with high-dose dexamethasone starting at 16 mg daily, and reducing to the lowest dose that keeps the patient symptom free.

Any general measure for improving well-being (e.g. correcting anaemia) will help.

Prescribe appropriately for any associated itch.

Seek a surgical opinion about the possibility of relieving biliary obstruction by stenting if the patient is fit for the procedure.

E Extra information

The results of chemotherapy and radiotherapy to relieve jaundice in palliative care are usually disappointing.

The patient and family members need to be sensitively informed about the poor prognosis, and offered appropriate support and reassurance that everything reasonable and possible will be done to relieve the itch and other symptoms. Changes in skin colour can develop and progress very rapidly and may be alarming, especially to younger members of the family.

Further reading

- Thorns A, Edmonds P. The management of pruritus in palliative care patients. *Eur J Palliat Care.* 2000; **7:** 9–12.

Chapter 38

Lymphoedema

> There is no one-to-one correlation between a disease and the spectrum of disability problems that may be associated with it.
>
> Walter Stolov[1]

Introduction

Lymphoedema is the accumulation of lymph in the soft tissues, secondary to a disruption in lymphatic drainage.

The most commonly seen situation is lymphoedema of the arm following lymph node dissection and radiotherapy for breast cancer, with an incidence of about 40%. This can develop at any time, from immediately following surgery to a few years later.

Lower limb oedema may occur in patients who have had inguinal lymph node dissections for intrapelvic tumours.

C Consider

Pathophysiology of lymphoedema

Lymph node damage by surgery and/or radiotherapy results in reduced drainage of fluid and protein from the distal parts of the affected limb.

Protein-rich fluid gathers in the limb, which stimulates the activity of fibroblasts, resulting in fibrosis.

The resulting 'brawny' tissues further strangle the lymphatics, resulting in overfilling of the remaining lymphatic vessels, which become engorged.

The lymph channel valves become damaged, causing further inhibition of normal drainage and even more fibrosis, and a vicious cycle of damage results.

Think about the possible causes of lymphoedema:

- abdominal or pelvic masses
- breast surgery (e.g. mastectomy involving block dissection of the axilla)
- radiotherapy, causing fibrosis
- tumour recurrence.

When did the swelling start in relation to surgery or radiotherapy? If the involved limb has been normal for a considerable time following treatment, think about the possibility of a recurrence of the tumour.

It is important to distinguish between simple oedema and lymphoedema. The main differences are summarised in the table overleaf.

	Simple oedema	*Lymphoedema*
Diuretics	Good response	Poor response
Elevation	Good response	Poor response
Limb affected	Usually lower and bilateral	Unilateral, often upper
Pressure	Pitting	Usually no pitting (due to fibrosis)
Skin	Tight, smooth	Hyperkeratotic

A Assess

Look for the following:

- blisters – 'lymph blisters' or lymphangiomas
- bruises (especially on the legs)
- deepening of the skin creases
- fungal infection
- inflammation
- Stemmer's sign (thickened skin at the bases of digits that cannot be pinched between the finger and thumb)
- ulcers (their presence indicates an additional venous disorder or cutaneous tumour deposits)
- weeping (lymphorrhoea).

The protein-rich fluid in lymphoedema is an excellent culture medium for bacteria, so the tiniest skin lesion represents a risk.

℞ Remedy

Lymphoedema is a complex problem that requires the input of several professionals.

The issues that need to be addressed will be considered in several broad categories.

Activities of daily living

Domestic work

Teach and reinforce the adoption of safe practices in the kitchen, such as the use of devices to aid one-handed work or reduce the risk of cuts and grazes to the affected limb.

Home environment

Liaise with occupational therapists with regard to the provision of equipment to make moving around at home easier (e.g. powered leg lifters to assist with getting into bed, powered bath hoists, powered recliner/self-lift chairs).

Self-care

The patient may require long-handled devices to assist with washing and drying if bending is restricted. Demonstrate to the patient and/or the carer the use of devices designed for getting compression sleeves or hosiery on and off.

Clothes

Advise about suitable clothing, including styles that are easy to put on and take off, or adapting existing clothing to give more room with the use of additional fastenings, etc.

Occasionally circumstances may require you to explain the use of some form of sling support for a grossly oedematous arm, or incorporation of some type of 'pocket' or 'apron' for the patient to use when moving around.

Compression and massage

Massage is carried out on dry skin, without lubricants, and the limb is gently massaged to aid the flow of lymph back towards the trunk.

Compression bandages or garments are applied afterwards to prevent re-accumulation of fluid in the limb, and these should be worn day and night. Exercises may be helpful for encouraging the lymph flow, and the affected joints should be exercised through their full range of movement at least twice every day. The limb should *not* be immobilised.

The affected limb should be elevated when resting. The arms should be raised to shoulder height by using pillows. The legs should be raised, when sitting, at least level with the hips. The foot of the bed can be raised at night by 2 to 3 inches.

Bandages must be kept clean and dry and must be washed and dried regularly.

Compression pumps are only used in specific instances and after assessment by suitably qualified professionals.

Drugs

Drug treatment is likely to be disappointing, but is possibly worth trying.

- Diuretics – furosemide 40 mg and spironolactone 100 mg in the morning can be tried for 3 days.
- Steroids should be tried if diuretics do not produce a result. Give dexamethasone 8 mg once in the morning, reducing the dose by 2 mg every third day. This is especially worth trying in cases of face, trunk or lower limb swelling, as the steroids may help to reduce the swelling around the tumour mass which is compressing the lymph channels.

Skin care

- Cleanliness is vitally important. Advise the use of a soap-free cleanser for the skin.
- Dry the skin carefully, paying special attention to the areas between the fingers and toes. Use a hairdryer set on a cool setting if necessary.
- Gloves must be used for gardening.
- Insect bites should be prevented if possible with repellent creams.
- Nail care is important, and special care must be taken when trimming the nails.
- Protect the limb from trauma as far as possible.
- Sunburn must be avoided.
- The affected limb must not be used for blood pressure measurements, injections or venepuncture, either for blood sampling or infusions.

Despite all the care and caution that the patient may exercise, infection is always a risk.

Always be on the alert for signs of infection, and treat with phenoxymethylpenicillin (500 mg 6-hourly) or erythromycin (500 mg 6-hourly) for 1 week, then continuing on half this dose for at least 6 weeks.

For patients who have repeated episodes of infection, long-term prophylactic phenoxymethylpenicillin (500 mg daily for 1 year) is the best way of preventing recurrent attacks and minimising infection-induced fibrosis.

E Extra information

Soaking dressings in copious amounts of normal saline prior to removal can reduce the risk of bleeding on removing dressings. Alternatively, soak the dressings off while the patient is in the bath.

To minimise the time for which the limb is left undressed (with a consequent risk of infection), all staff involved in reviewing the patient's progress should liaise with each other and agree suitable times for assessing the limb.

Be aware of the distress to patients and their relatives that is associated with changes in body image and feelings of revulsion at enlarged distorted heavy limbs.

Reference

1 Stolov W. Evaluation of the patient. In: *Krusen's Handbook of Physical Medicine and Rehabilitation.* Philadelphia, PA: WB Saunders; 1990.

Further reading

- Diegan M. Self-sufficiency the aim in lymphoedema care. *Forum.* 2005; **December:** 37–8.
- Hardy D. Managing long-term conditions: non-cancer-related lymphoedema.*Br J Nursing.* 2006; **15:** 444–52.
- Twycross R, Jenns K, Todd J. *Lymphoedema.* Oxford: Radcliffe Medical Press; 2000.

Chapter 39

Mouth problems

> In damp places there grow tiny creatures too small for us to see, which make their way into our bodies through the mouth and nose and give rise to grave illnesses.
>
> Marcus Varro (Roman physician, first century BC), *De Re Rustica*

Introduction

Dry mouth (xerostomia) is a common condition, affecting around 40% of hospice patients but probably affecting most cancer patients at some stage as a result of treatment and general poor health.

A sore mouth is most commonly due to candida infection, which occurs in about 10–15% of patients with cancer at almost any stage of the illness. The incidence in terminally ill patients is probably nearer 90%.

C Consider

- Concurrent disease (e.g. uncontrolled diabetes).
- Drugs – anticholinergics, antihistamines, anticonvulsants, beta-blockers, diuretics, opioids or steroids (which predispose to candida infection).
- Hypercalcaemia.
- Inadequate fluid intake causing dehydration.
- Malnutrition (e.g. anaemia, protein deficiency or vitamin deficiency).
- Mouth breathing, either by day due to debility or when asleep.
- Mucositis secondary to chemotherapy.
- Oral infection (e.g. candida).
- Oxygen therapy.
- Radiotherapy to the head and neck causing diminution of salivary secretion.

A Assess

Ask about the following:

- antibiotics – antibiotic treatment increases the risk of oral candidiasis
- bleeding
- chemotherapy given recently – the epithelial cells of the oral mucosa have a rapid proliferation rate which renders them very susceptible to chemotherapy
- dental problems
- dentures that don't fit well
- difficulty in chewing or swallowing
- drugs currently being taken
- dryness
- pain
- radiotherapy to the head and neck at any time
- smoking
- taste alteration.

A lot can be learned from an examination of the mouth, and one does not have to be a dentist!

Breath

Check for halitosis and think about what the smell of the breath might indicate (*see* Chapter 33 on halitosis for further details).

Lips

Look for cheilosis, cracked dry lips and evidence of infection such as herpes.

Oral cavity

- *Dentures*. Do they fit well? Are they clean? Ask the patient to remove them, and then look at the gums and palate where infection could be lurking.
- *Gums*. Is there gingivitis or evidence of bleeding or abrasion from dentures?
- *Hard and soft palate*. Look for lesions, including infection and leucoplakia. Candida scrapes off, whereas leucoplakia does not.
- *Mucosa*. Look for candida and ulceration, including aphthous ulcers.
- *Teeth*. Look for decay, rough and broken edges and signs of infection.
- *Tongue*. Look for fissures, coating and evidence of infection, the state of the papillae and how moist the tongue is.

Assess the patient's general health, looking at the following:

- their general condition and ability to attend to their oral hygiene
- hydration and their ability to maintain a reasonable oral fluid intake
- their nutritional state.

℞ Remedy

General measures

Assess the mouth every day. Infections start quickly and are easily overlooked.
Deal with any general issues that may require attention.

- *Dentures*. Do they need to be adjusted, relined or remade?
- *Drugs*. These include antidepressants, cyclizine, diuretics, hyoscine and opioids.
- *Fluid intake*. Encourage intake of small regular amounts of fluid orally if possible
- *Food*. Taste, temperature, texture and moistness.
- *Fluoride*. Fluoride mouthwashes or fluoride gel at night helps to protect the vulnerable areas of the teeth around the gum margins. Alcohol-free mouthwashes are least stinging. Toothpaste with a higher fluoride content marketed under the trade name 'Duraphat' and manufactured by Colgate is available on prescription, but at the time of writing (September 2006) is not yet available over the counter.
- *Ice cubes or frozen fruit segments*. These can be sucked to keep the mouth moist.
- *Infection*. Candida, or herpes simplex following chemotherapy.
- *Oral hygiene*.
- *Pineapple chunks*. These contain ananase, which helps to clean the mouth.

- *Saliva.* Does the patient need an artificial saliva spray to keep the mouth moist and comfortable?

Involving the family

The patient and their family can be involved in the following measures.

- *Artificial saliva.* Frequent sprays of 'artificial saliva' may help some patients. Several artificial saliva aerosol sprays are available on prescription.
- *Bicarbonate of soda mouthwashes.* Use half a teaspoonful of bicarbonate to 300 ml of lukewarm water. These mouthwashes help to loosen debris and are soothing. Advise the patient not to swallow.
- *Chilled fruit.* Chilled fruit jellies, ice lollipops, or chilled slivers of pineapple to suck (discard the residue). Tinned pineapple in natural juice is preferable to fresh fruit.
- *Ice.* Iced water or a dish of crushed ice with a spoon to serve small amounts.
- *Juices.* Fresh orange, lemon or grapefruit juice, although this may sting.
- *Moistening the mouth.* If the patient is very poorly, a few drips of water from a syringe may help to keep the mouth moist and make the patient more comfortable.
- *Pineapple chunks.* Pineapple contains a proteolytic enzyme, ananase, which also cleans the mouth. The tinned variety, in natural fruit juice rather than syrup, is better tolerated than fresh pineapple, and can be more easily stored and used.
- *Sparkling water.* Tonic or soda water may be tried, either chilled or frozen as ice cubes.
- *Yogurt.* Either chilled or frozen, this soothes a sore mouth.

Specific measures

Aphthous ulcers

Hydrocortisone pellets (2.5 mg four times daily), corticosteroids in lozenges or in paste, followed by carmellose gelatin paste.

Candidiasis

Topical nystatin suspension (2 ml four times a day) or miconazole gel (5–10 ml four times daily, held in the mouth with dentures removed). Resistant candidiasis usually responds to systemic oral fluconazole (50 mg capsule daily for 7–14 days).

When treating candida or other mouth infections, particular attention should be paid to dentures to ensure that they do not harbour infection. Similarly, toothbrushes should be renewed after any oral infection.

Mouth pain

- Benzocaine/cetalkonium aerosol (AAA spray) may help to relieve the pain of a malignant ulcer of the mouth or tonsil.
- Benzydamine 0.15% oral rinse or gargle, 15 ml every 1 to 2 hours, will help painful inflammation of the mouth and throat, including ulceration.
- Carbenoxolone 2% gel or triamcinolone 0.1% in Orabase cream may also be used to treat mouth ulcers.

Mucositis

Sucralfate is useful for the management of mucositis. Rinse the suspension round the mouth for 2 minutes, and then swallow. Alternatively, crush one tablet and spread round the mouth. If the mouth is dry, the tablet can be mixed in a sterile lubricating jelly (e.g. KY Jelly). Do this after meals and at bedtime.

Post-radiation xerostomia

Try pilocarpine 5–7.5 mg three or four times a day.

E Extra information

Candidiasis is the commonest cause of oral infection, and is usually obvious as a raw oral mucosa coated with white plaques, but candidiasis in the mouth may present as redness alone without the white plaques.

Aphthous ulcers are much less common than oral candidiasis.

Mouthwashes containing glycerin are not recommended, as they actually dry the oral mucosa over a period of time.

Further reading

- Bagg J. Oral candidosis: how to treat a common problem. *Eur J Palliat Care.* 2003; **10:** 54–6.
- Coulter S, Gray R, Watson M. The need for dental involvement in palliative care. *Eur J Palliat Care.* 2006; **13:** 94–7.
- Flint S. Oral ulceration: GP guide to diagnosis and treatment. *Prescriber.* 2005; **17:** 32–48.
- Mercadante S. Dry mouth and palliative care. *Eur J Palliat Care.* 2002; **9:** 182–5.

Chapter 40

Nausea and vomiting

> I eat to live, to serve and also, if it so happens, to enjoy, but I do not eat for the sake of enjoyment.
>
> Mahatama Gandhi (1869–1948)

Introduction

Nausea and vomiting are two symptoms that are very distressing to both the patient and their relatives.

Nausea is the unpleasant feeling of needing to vomit, and may be accompanied by symptoms such as feeling sweaty and clammy, and the patient may have no desire to do anything except lie quiet and still.

Vomiting is the forceful expulsion of the gastric contents through the mouth.

Many patients can tolerate a couple of episodes of vomiting a day, especially if it brings relief of their symptoms, but persistent nausea causes misery which many find intolerable and very debilitating.

Nausea is under the physiological control of the vomiting centre in the medulla. This in turn is under the influence of higher centres in the brain – the vestibular nuclei and the chemoreceptor trigger zone (CTZ) in the floor of the fourth ventricle.

C Consider

The causes of nausea and vomiting in cancer include the following:

- ascites
- brain metastases
- cough
- drugs – for example:
  - antibiotics
  - NSAIDs
  - opioids
- gastrointestinal causes:
  - bowel obstruction
  - constipation
  - gastric stasis
  - gastritis
  - oropharyngeal candidiasis
- metabolic disturbances:
  - hypercalcaemia
  - septicaemia
  - uraemia
- pain
- psychosomatic causes – fear and anxiety
- toxins:
  - chemotherapy

- — infections
- — paraneoplastic syndromes
- — radiotherapy.

A Assess

Nausea and vomiting should be assessed separately.

It is essential to distinguish between cough with expectoration, regurgitation and true vomiting.

What is the pattern of the nausea? Is it intermittent or persistent? Is it of recent onset? Is nausea accompanied by hiccupping or retching? Are there prolonged times after vomiting when the patient is relatively or completely symptom free?

Are there any other symptoms, such as headache, associated with the vomiting?

What is the likely extent of the patient's disease? Does this explain the patient's nausea?

Review the medications. Did the nausea start after introducing a new drug treatment?

Assess the vomitus. Does it contain undigested food, faecal content or blood?

Conduct a general examination, including the cranial nerves and the optic fundi for papilloedema (cerebral metastases), and a rectal examination if constipation is suspected. An empty but ballooned rectum indicates a higher faecal obstruction.

Check blood urea, electrolytes and calcium.

℞ Remedy

Explain the likely cause and the management plan to the patient.

Consider simple measures such as dietary advice.

Non-pharmacological management of nausea and vomiting

- Remove food from sight and keep cooking smells to a minimum.
- Only offer foods that are tolerated and that the patient likes, and offer small portions.
- Patients at home who are self-caring may benefit from having someone else cook food so that they can avoid the aromas of food cooking. Here are some ideas that have been tried and tested:
  - — when cooking cabbage or sprouts, a small bay leaf or a slice of bread added to the water greatly reduces the cooking smell. Rye bread is particularly effective
  - — the smell of cauliflower cooking can be reduced by adding lemon to the saucepan. Half of the 'shell' of a squeezed lemon can be used
  - — the smell of fish cooking can be minimised by adding celery stalks or leaves to the saucepan. A fishy smell on the dishes is easily removed by adding a spoonful of vinegar to the washing-up water
  - — burning a candle near the cooker can reduce cooking smells in the kitchen. Remind the patient not to leave it unattended!
- Patients who wish to avoid taking medicines may wish to try wrist acupressure bands, which are commercially available.
- Unpleasant odours (e.g. from a fungating wound) may be partially responsible and should be controlled if possible.

Relevant physiology and pharmacology

Several neurotransmitter receptors, which respond to a variety of stimuli, are responsible for patients feeling nauseated. Various emetic stimuli result in impulses being relayed to the vomiting centre in the medulla and the CTZ in the floor of the fourth ventricle. The neurotransmitter receptors involved include those for histamine, acetylcholine, dopamine and 5HT.

The patient's nausea may be caused by more than one stimulus activating more than one site in the brain. As a result, on some occasions more than one drug may be required for symptom control. Oral medication may be adequate to control nausea, but the rectal or subcutaneous route may be better for persistent nausea.

Levomepromazine antagonises several receptors. This makes it a useful drug in cases where the cause of the nausea is unclear, or while awaiting the results of blood tests to determine the precise cause. It may be a useful single agent at a starting dose of 6.25 mg once or twice daily, and can be given orally or by injection. Higher doses may be sedative.

Anti-emetics should be given regularly at first. When the cause of the vomiting has been addressed, they may be used on an 'as required' basis.

Antihistamines (cyclizine)

The vomiting centre has many histamine and acetylcholine receptors. Cyclizine is an antihistamine anti-emetic that also has antimuscarinic actions, so its side-effects include a dry mouth.

Antimuscarinics (hyoscine hydrobromide)

Hyoscine hydrobromide is a potent antimuscarinic and is especially useful for colic associated with bowel obstruction.

Antipsychotics (haloperidol, prochlorperazine, levomepromazine)

Drugs and metabolic upsets both cause nausea by stimulating receptors in the CTZ. The antipsychotics act as powerful dopamine inhibitors, and are effective in controlling nausea due to these causes.

Levomepromazine has antimuscarinic, antihistamine, anxiolytic and $5HT_2$-antagonist effects, making it a broad-spectrum anti-emetic at low doses.

Prokinetics (metoclopramide, domperidone)

Metoclopramide acts peripherally on the gut to restore normal gastric emptying, and also on the CTZ, which means that it crosses the blood–brain barrier and may have a role in drug-induced nausea.

Domperidone is similar to metoclopramide but does not cross the blood–brain barrier.

$5HT_3$ antagonists (ondansetron, granisetron)

The $5HT_3$ receptors are located in the CTZ and are particularly responsive to stimuli produced by radiotherapy and chemotherapy. Ondansetron or granisetron are the drugs of choice for nausea due to this cause.

Steroids

Corticosteroids are not anti-emetics as such, but sometimes have a non-specific action in reducing nausea and vomiting and, of course, have a role in reducing

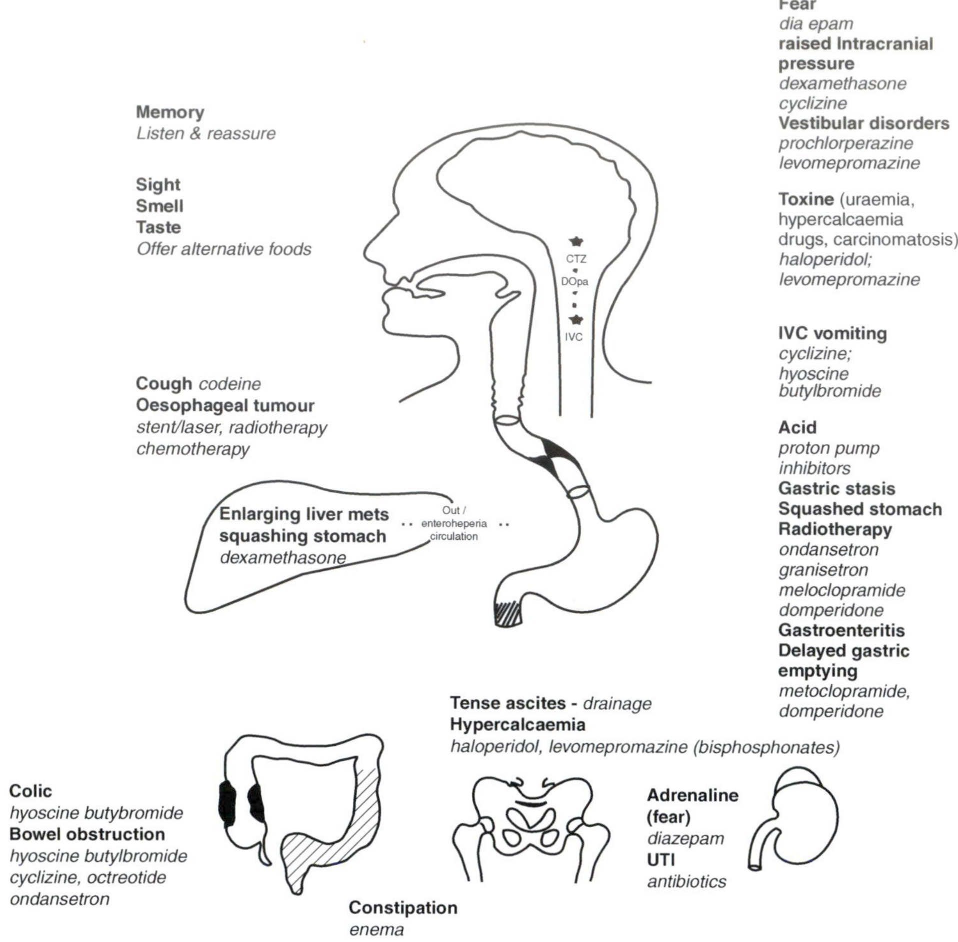

Figure 40.1 Summary of the main causes and treatments of nausea and vomiting.

raised intracranial pressure or reducing the size of an enlarging liver pressing on the stomach.

Pharmacological management of specific causes of nausea and vomiting

Treat any specific and reversible causes of nausea and vomiting, such as pain, cough or infection. The choice of an effective anti-emetic depends on the reason for the nausea and vomiting. The first thing to do is to establish the cause and look at the pathophysiology of the problem. Then, by applying pharmacology, an effective solution can be reached.

- *Constipation.* An empty ballooned rectum indicates a higher faecal obstruction. Use enemas to clear the lower bowel, and regular laxatives to prevent recurrence, especially if the patient is on opioids.
- *Gastritis.* Epigastric tenderness and discomfort may be due to gastric irritation from NSAIDs, which should be stopped. If these are not the cause, consider

using a proton pump inhibitor to relieve the discomfort, and either cyclizine 50 mg three times a day or ondansetron 8 mg twice daily.

- *Hypercalcaemia*. This usually presents with associated confusion and dehydration. Haloperidol 1.5 mg once or twice daily, or levomepromazine 6.25 mg as a starting dose should relieve the nausea, and the patient should be rehydrated with IV fluids and the hypercalcaemia corrected with bisphosphonates.
- *Intestinal obstruction*. Assuming that surgery is not an option and palliation of symptoms is the goal, try one of the following drugs:
  - — cyclizine 150 mg per 24 hours SC or orally
  - — hyoscine butylbromide 40–100 mg per 24 hours SC
  - — octreotide 300–1000 μg per 24hours SC
  - — ondansetron 8–24 mg per 24 hours orally, IV or SC.
- *Opioid-induced vomiting*. Opioids cause vomiting by a combination of mechanisms, including stimulation of the CTZ, increased vestibular sensitivity, gastric stasis and reduced intestinal motility. The latter results in constipation. Gastric stasis responds to metoclopramide, but the usual first-line treatments for opioid-induced vomiting are haloperidol, cyclizine or hyoscine hydrobromide.
- *Oropharyngeal candidiasis*. Treat with either nystatin or fluconazole until the infection is completely cleared.
- *Raised intracranial pressure*. Cyclizine 50 mg three times daily by mouth or 150 mg per 24 hours SC should control the vomiting, and dexamethasone 4–16 mg per 24 hours (given in the morning) will help to reduce the pressure and further relieve symptoms. Doses should be reviewed as the patient improves and depending on whether the cause of the raised pressure can be treated.
- *Urinary tract infection*. Treat with appropriate antibiotics, recognising that some of these may also cause nausea.

E Extra information

The presence of nausea offers a good opportunity to review the patient's medication and discontinue as many drugs as possible in case they are causing the nausea. It is also an ideal time to review the opioid dose.

Anti-emetics may be administered rectally or possibly via a syringe driver, which avoids the risk of them being lost the next time the patient vomits.

With the exception of pain, nausea that prohibits eating upsets the family more than any other symptom, so it is important to review the patient regularly. Be sure to explain that nausea associated with opioids is short-lived, and tolerance will develop in a few days.

Nausea and vomiting in cancer often have more than one cause. For this reason a second anti-emetic is often required.

If you are reasonably sure that a single factor is responsible, choose the anti-emetic that is most likely to help first time:

- cerebral tumours – cyclizine
- drug and metabolic causes – haloperidol
- gastric stasis – metoclopramide
- intestinal obstruction – cyclizine.

If the cause is not reasonably clear, try haloperidol, cyclizine or levomepromazine.

If combined anti-emetics are required, use drugs with different modes of action (*see* section on relevant physiology and pharmacology, p. 173).

Haloperidol and cyclizine are a reasonable combination to start with. Because cyclizine can antagonise the prokinetic effects of metoclopramide, these two drugs should not usually be mixed.

Levomepromazine acts at several receptor sites and may be a useful single agent, or may replace a combination that has been tried and which has proved unsuccessful.

Some patients might wish to try complementary therapies, including acupuncture or acupressure or other complementary therapy, such as hypnosis and imagery.

Further reading

- Anon. Datafile on nausea and vomiting. *Prescriber.* 2005; **16**: 68–9.
- Fallon R, Fraser C, Moriarty K. Recommended management of nausea and vomiting. *Prescriber.* 2005; **16:** 57–67.
- Perdue C. Understanding nausea and vomiting in advanced cancer. *Nurs Times.* 2005; **101:** 32–5.

Chapter 41

Nightmares

> The surgeon knows all the parts of the brain but he does not know his patient's dreams.
>
> Richard Selzer, US surgeon[1]

Introduction

The *Oxford Dictionary* defines a nightmare as a frightening dream. It gives the etymology of the word as follows: 'Old English mære incubus (evil spirit), once thought to lie on and suffocate sleepers'.

Nightmares are the body's way of expressing fear, and it may help for the patient to share the nightmare and 'externalise' that fear and seek appropriate reassurance and help.

C Consider

What does the patient mean by 'nightmares'? The word has assumed a wider meaning than the one given above, and may be used to describe a recurring dream or situation that is hard to cope with. The patient is almost certainly facing a very anxious time in their life, so to offer the appropriate help, one needs to know what the patient is experiencing.

It is important to think about the different types of events that the patient may experience.

Hallucinations

Hallucinations are disorders of perception. They may be visual, auditory, tactile or olfactory in nature, and they occur in the absence of a corresponding external stimulus.

There are two different types of hallucinations:

- hypnagogic hallucinations, which occur when falling asleep. This term describes the occurrence of visions or dreams during the drowsy state following sleep [Greek *hypnos* (sleep) and *agbgos* (leading)]
- hypnopompic hallucinations, which occur when waking. This denotes the occurrence of visions or dreams during the drowsy state following sleep [Greek *hypnos* (sleep) and *pompe* (procession)].

Both are normal and usually simple (e.g. hearing a telephone or doorbell, or hearing one's name being called).

Illusions

An illusion is a false perception of a real object or a misinterpretation of an actual stimulus (e.g. mistaking a nurse for a relative).

Nightmares

A nightmare is an unpleasant or frightening dream that occurs during rapid-eye-movement (REM) sleep. The content of a dream or nightmare may be very significant. It can indicate fears or anxieties that the patient is unable to express while awake.

Night terrors

Night terrors are common in children, but uncommon in adults. They occur at a different point of the sleep cycle from nightmares, and are accompanied by considerable autonomic and motor disturbance.

A Assess

- What exactly is the patient describing?
- How bad is the problem?
- Are these nightmares occurring every night and disrupting sleep?
- When did these nightmares start?
- How frequent are they?
- Is the subject or content the same every night?
- Does the patient feel the same fear or sensation during the day?
- Is there a relationship between the onset and a new event or a change in medication?
- Find out the part that drugs may play in the patient's nightmares.
- How does the patient see their future?
- Have they talked about dying or do they fear the process of dying?
- What clues did this discu0ssion reveal about any fears that the patient may be experiencing?

℞ Remedy

Build a relationship with the patient, based on trust, caring and empathy. This will help the patient to air their fears and anxieties.

Explore any anxieties with the patient and deal with anything that arises, offering appropriate counselling or arranging a visit from a minister of religion or a spiritual needs adviser as appropriate.

Discontinue or adjust the doses of any causative drugs. Reduce the dose of opioids if possible.

Prescribe a neuroleptic drug, such as haloperidol (0.5–5 mg at night), when necessary.

Seek the help of a psychiatrist for true hallucinations not associated with drugs.

E Extra information

Drugs may interfere with sleep patterns. Any of the following drugs may contribute to nightmares:

- alcohol
- anticholinergic drugs

- caffeine
- hypnotics
- tricyclic antidepressants.

Withdrawal of alcohol or sedatives may do likewise. Has the patient been deprived of a regular alcohol intake since admission to hospital?

Reference

1 Selzer R. *Mortal Lessons*. London: Chatto & Windus; 1981. p. 21.

Further reading

No relevant journal papers were identified.

Chapter 42

Opioid-induced sedation

> Opium, used internally, acts as a very powerful stimulant, then as a sedative, and finally as an anodyne and narcotic.
>
> Anon.[1]

Introduction

Some patients associate morphine with the end stages of their illness and expect it to cause drowsiness. They mistakenly assume that starting opioids means that they can no longer expect to be alert, take part in conversation, read the newspaper, etc. These concerns need to be addressed and any expressed misconceptions corrected.

C Consider

There are several possible reasons why a patient becomes drowsy. One of these is an excessive dose of opioids, but there are others that must be considered.

Think about the opioid prescription.

- Is the pain opioid-sensitive? An *excess* of opioid can certainly cause sedation, and doses must be titrated to response.
- Has the opioid dose been increased recently? Did the drowsiness start after that?
- Has the patient accidentally taken too much of their medication?
- Has the patient's condition and their ability to metabolise morphine deteriorated?
- Has the pain been relieved by another means (e.g. a nerve block), which has resulted in a reduction in the opioid dose needed?

Think about other causes of drowsiness.

- Is the patient also on a sedative?
- Centrally acting anti-emetic drugs such as cyclizine and haloperidol, or amitriptyline given for nerve pain, could be partly to blame.
- Has anything been obtained 'over the counter' that could have caused a drug interaction or be causing drowsiness?
- Does the patient have known or suspected renal impairment?
- Are there any factors in the patient's clinical condition that are likely to cause sedation, such as hypercalcaemia?
- Has the patient deteriorated?

A Assess

The sedative effect of opioid drugs is normally short-lived. The effect will be aggravated by the concomitant use of other sedative drugs, such as benzodiazepines.

Establish the doses of drugs that are being prescribed and the duration of treatment. Are immediate-release or modified-release preparations being used?

Check that the prescribed dose is the dose that the patient has actually received.

Review all of the other drugs that are being prescribed.

The clearance of morphine is not affected by impaired renal function, but accumulation of morphine glucuronides occurs. It is likely that accumulation of morphine-6-glucuronide is responsible for the increased toxicity effects of morphine in patients with renal failure.

Check renal function and corrected serum calcium concentration.

℞ Remedy

Reduce or stop any other sedative drugs that are being prescribed.

If the patient's pain is controlled, omit the next dose of morphine and reduce subsequent doses appropriately. Fentanyl skin patches have a long half-life and will take longer to 'wash out' of the body, and this should be explained to the patient's family.

Prescribe an appropriate breakthrough dose of analgesia to be used in the event of pain.

Consider the use of adjuvants for the control of pain.

Consider the use of non-drug measures, such as radiotherapy.

Where possible and appropriate, correct any metabolic abnormalities.

Review the patient regularly and adjust opioid doses according to the patient's response.

E Extra information

Sedation is a very common side-effect of opioid drugs. Most patients develop selective tolerance to the effects of opioid drugs, with the exception of analgesia and constipation. If a patient has been maintained on a dose of an opioid, one would expect the sedative effect to diminish after 48–72 hours. If the dose of opioid is escalated rapidly, sedation will be a greater problem. The sedative effect of drugs used in combination may be additive (e.g. benzodiazepines, cyclizine and carbamazepine).

It is rarely necessary to use drugs such as naloxone which antagonise the effects of morphine.

Reference

1 Anon. Entry number 700. In: *Enquire Within Upon Everything*. London: Houlston and Sons; 1890.

Further reading

No relevant journal papers were identified.

Chapter 43

Skin at risk of ulceration

Woollen clothing keeps the skin healthy.

Venetian proverb

Introduction

Over the years, a number of terms have been used to describe damage to the skin associated with immobility, impaired circulation and poor health resulting in prolonged immobility. The term 'bed sores' is not accurate. 'Decubitus ulcer' is not necessarily accurate either, since the Latin word *'decub'* translates as 'lying down', and many of these lesions develop while the patient is sitting in a chair. We shall therefore use the term 'pressure ulcer'.

The term 'pressure ulcer' is defined by the European Pressure Ulcer Advisory Panel as 'an area of localised damage to the skin and underlying tissue caused by pressure, shear or friction, or a combination of these'.[1]

C Consider

Pressure ulcers can occur in any patient who is immobile for long periods. To assess the risk to an individual, it is essential to understand the way in which ulcers develop.

Pathogenesis of pressure ulcers

There are four main factors that contribute to the development of pressure ulcers:

- friction
- moisture
- pressure
- shear.

It is important to bear these in mind when considering the factors that put the patient at risk of skin trauma.

Friction

Friction between the skin and another surface can result in the development of small intradermal blisters which in turn lead to superficial breaks in the skin surface. This can either initiate or speed up the development of a pressure ulcer.

Moisture

Moisture causes maceration and softening of the skin, and increases the damaging effects of friction up to fivefold.

Pressure

Pressure can be tolerated for short periods, and when it is removed there is a reactive increase in blood flow, resulting in local redness.

Sustained pressure results in the following chain of events:

1 decreased capillary flow
2 ischaemia, localised small thrombus formation and lymphatic occlusion
3 increased capillary permeability
4 entry of fluid into the extravascular space, causing oedema
5 cell death and tissue death.

These changes can affect the skin, subcutaneous tissues or superficial muscle.

Shear

Shearing force is generated by motion between underlying bone and the subcutaneous tissues. Basically the skin remains static with respect to the sheet, and the bone moves underneath. Anything that results in increased shearing forces (including tilting the bed by more than about 30° above the horizontal) increases the risk of damage. Tilting the bed dramatically reduces the pressure required to cause localised ischaemia.

Consider the other factors that might be putting your patient at risk of a pressure ulcer. These include the following:

- anaemia
- cachexia
- dressings, clothing or bandages causing abrasion
- hypoproteinaemia causing interstitial oedema
- immobility of any part due to any cause
- immunosuppression, which increases the risk of infection
- malnutrition and vitamin C or zinc deficiency, which impair wound healing
- neurological deficit (e.g. diabetes)
- restraints or rails that could cause injury or pressure
- steroids given long term impair healing and increase infection risk
- vascular insufficiency
- wet skin.

A Assess

Assess the patient's degree of risk from the factors listed above, and deal with and correct as many of these as possible.

Use a validated assessment tool (e.g. Waterlow score) to quantify risk.

℞ Remedy

Prevention

Prevention, if possible, is the aim. There are four main areas to look at:

- general measures
- nutrition
- pressure redistribution
- skin care.

General measures

- Clean, dry skin must be maintained at all times.
- Mobilise the patient as much as possible with passive exercises if they are immobile.
- Pressure relief so that blood supply is not impaired.
- Protection against trauma and reinfection.
- Sitting out of bed if possible.

Nutrition

- Balanced diet to ensure adequate protein and vitamin intake.
- Iron to correct anaemia if required.
- Serum albumin kept within normal limits to prevent interstitial oedema.
- Vitamin C 500–1000 mg daily if indicated.
- Zinc supplements if necessary.

Pressure redistribution

- Elbow and heel protection.
- Frequent movement and repositioning should be encouraged in patients who can move independently.
- Frequent repositioning is necessary for dependent patients.
- Mattress most appropriate to the patient's needs and weight.
- Wheelchair cushion.

Skin care

- Dry skin should be moisturised.
- Moist skin (due to urine, faeces or discharges) should be cleaned, dried and protected.
- Remove restraints and bed rails where possible to prevent injury.
- Reposition the patient frequently and check the skin each time.
- Tilting above 30° should be avoided if possible.

Treatment

General measures

Aim for the maximum improvement possible in the patient's general health and nutritional state. Treat pain and discomfort and help the patient to cope with the psychological impact of having a pressure ulcer that might never heal.

Specific measures

- Debridement of any pus and dead material from the wound surface.
- Exudate and odour should be managed with appropriate dressings.
- Infection management with appropriate antibiotics.
- Protect vulnerable skin and granulating tissues.

E Extra information

Almost 20% of pressure ulcers occur in patients who are being cared for at home. Regular assessment by a trained person is vital, and should be arranged and carried out by the community nurse.

Time is well spent in educating the family about prevention. They can be taught about the following:

- lifting the patient to avoid shearing forces on body tissues, rather than pushing or pulling
- pillows to support the body and to separate the areas of contact
- pressure-relieving interventions
- regularly repositioning the patient.

Ring cushions are advertised in many of the magazines that offer aids for disabled people. Make the patient and family aware that these can compromise the circulation and should not be used.

Sheepskins are useful complements to other support systems. They keep the skin dry and reduce friction. Make sure that the family carers are aware that sheepskins do not relieve pressure.

Reference

1 European Pressure Ulcer Advisory Panel. *Pressure Ulcer Prevention Guidelines;* www.epuap.org/glprevention.html

Further reading

- Grey JE, Enoch S, Harding KG. Pressure ulcers (in ABC of wound healing). *BMJ.* 2006; **332:** 472–5.
- Iglesias C, Nixon J, Cranny G *et al.* Pressure-relieving support surfaces (PRESSURE) trial: cost-effectiveness analysis. *BMJ.* 2006; **332:** 1416–18.
- Nixon J, Cranny G, Iglesias C *et al.* Randomised controlled trial of alternating pressure mattresses compared with alternating pressure overlays for the prevention of pressure ulcers: PRESSURE (pressure-relieving support surfaces) trial. *BMJ.* 2006; **332:** 1413–15.
- Vale L, Noble DW. Overlays or mattresses to prevent pressure sores? *BMJ.* 2006; **332:** 1401–2.
- Zeppetella G. Topical opioids for painful skin ulcers: do they work? *Eur J Palliat Care.* 2004; **11:** 93–6.

Chapter 44

Sleep disorders

Sleep is the only medicine that gives ease.

Sophocles (*c*.496–406 BC), *Philocetes 766*

Introduction

Many patients in palliative care settings complain of tiredness and fatigue, and many attribute this to poor sleep. They may experience difficulty in getting to sleep, difficulty in staying asleep, wakening early, waking normally but still feeling tired, or a combination of these.

C Consider

Sleep deprivation has several important outcomes:

- irritability
- loss of will due to exhaustion, resulting in inability to cope
- lowered pain threshold, resulting in worsening of pain which interferes with sleep, and the lack of sleep further reduces the pain threshold
- tiredness and reduced activity, which increases the risk of pressure ulcers.

A Assess

Explore with the patient what type of sleep problem they have (getting to sleep, early wakening, etc.).

Find out why the patient is not sleeping. Possible causes include the following:

- breathing difficulty, especially when lying down
- delirium, with a disturbed body rhythm
- depression
- fear (e.g. of dying while asleep)
- itch
- nausea and vomiting
- nightmares
- pain
- restless leg syndrome
- unfinished business and anxiety about this.

Think about prescribed drugs that could be responsible. These include the following:

- diuretics (given too late and causing nocturia)
- propranolol (can cause nightmares)
- steroids (especially if given after 6 pm)
- stimulant antidepressants (e.g. fluoxetine)
- theophyllines.

Ask about medications that are not being prescribed. Many patients buy additional products.

Check the following:

- alcohol intake
- caffeine intake
- tobacco use.

Have any of these changed since admission to the hospital or hospice?

Patients who are being cared for at home may be lying still with their eyes closed, appearing to be asleep, while in fact they are awake, alert and possibly agitated, but not wishing to disturb their carer, who needs their sleep, too, so that they can continue to offer care. If there appears to be a discrepancy in the reports given by the patient and their carer, investigate this possibility.

℞ Remedy

General and non-pharmacological measures

Attempt to re-establish the normal sleep/wake cycle by encouraging as much exercise and activity as possible and discouraging daytime napping.

Discourage the use of caffeine and cigarettes in the evening.

Let patients try the following simple measures to see whether they help:

- bathing in order to relax before going to bed
- massage or aromatherapy to aid relaxation
- music to aid relaxation and sleep
- progressive muscle relaxation
- warm milk or a carbohydrate snack at bedtime.

Pharmacological measures

- *Delirium with daytime sleeping.* Haloperidol 0.5–2.0 mg orally at teatime.
- *Depression.* Amitriptyline given 2 hours before bedtime is sedating.
- *Pain.* Opioids in a modified-release preparation.
- *Short-term insomnia with no specific cause.* Benzodiazepines.

Give diuretics and steroids as a single morning dose if possible.

E Extra information

Withdrawal of alcohol on admission may be the reason for disturbed sleep in hospital, but the patient may be reluctant to admit this. Ask about the withdrawal of other sedative drugs (e.g. benzodiazepines or even sleep aids bought over the counter).

Further reading

- Sanna P, Bruera E. Insomnia and sleep disturbances. *Eur J Palliat Care.* 2002; **9:** 8–12.

Chapter 45

Spinal cord compression

People of wealth and rank never use ugly names for ugly things. Apoplexy is an affection of the head: paralysis is nervousness: gangrene is pain and inconvenience in the extremities.

Sydney Smith (British churchman and essayist, 1771–1845)

Introduction

Spinal cord compression is seen in about 5% of cancer patients overall, with an incidence of about 15% in myeloma sufferers and around 10% in patients with prostate cancer.

It is an emergency, and symptoms can develop rapidly.

One of the dilemmas is whether to refer the patient for radiotherapy, as the results can be disappointing. If a long and difficult journey is required for radiotherapy treatment and the prognosis is short, it is essential to discuss, in clear unambiguous terms, the various options available and to consider the patient's priorities for their remaining time.

C Consider

The spinal column is the commonest site for bone secondary deposits. At autopsy, 70% of cancer patients will have a vertebral column deposit.

Lung, breast, lymphoma, myeloma and prostate primaries all metastasise to the spine, as do cancers from unknown primary sites. About two-thirds will occur in the thoracic spine and about a quarter in the lumbosacral spine. The majority will occur in the vertebral body, but some may invade the intervertebral foramen and compress the cord without involving the bony structures.

The symptoms probably arise from a combination of cord compression and involvement of the neighbouring blood supply.

The usual sequence of events is as follows:

1 pain, *progressing to*
2 weakness of the limbs with brisk reflexes and extensor plantar response, *progressing to*
3 sensory changes, *progressing to*
4 sphincter dysfunction.

The most important single prognostic guide is the level of neurological function at the beginning of treatment.

The rates of progression vary and can be either slow or very rapid.

Slow progression

Slow progression, with pain for several months before any neurological symptoms or signs develop, is typical of breast cancer and lymphomas.

Very rapid progression

In this case, the symptoms and signs develop over a period of a few hours and result in complete and irreversible cord damage. This is more likely to occur in lung cancer, myeloma and renal cancers.

A Assess

Pain is the presenting symptom in 95% of patients and the only symptom in about 10% of patients. The pain may be local or radicular.

Symptoms of compression

Local back pain

- Almost always present, usually midline or paravertebral in situation.
- Close to the lesion and well localised.
- Constant.
- Exacerbated by an increase in intrathoracic pressure (e.g. due to coughing or sneezing).
- Relieved by sitting or standing (the opposite of a vertebral disc lesion).

Radicular pain

- About two-thirds of patients experience radicular pain.
- Caused by compression of spinal roots.
- Incidence is about 90% of lumbosacral, 80% of cervical and 50% of thoracic metastases.
- Numbness and tingling may be present.
- Pain is improved by sitting and standing.
- Pain is worse at night.
- Radiation of pain is 'band-like' or girdle pain from back to front or usually unilateral and following the dermatome in the leg. The distribution of the pain can be used to localise the site of the lesion to the vertebral segment affected.
- Similar to pain from intervertebral disc disease, and should be distinguished from nerve plexus involvement.

Always be very suspicious when a patient reports back pain or pain in muscle or down a particular nerve distribution.

Encourage patients to report new pains promptly.

Vigilance and early diagnosis are essential. Ask about the following:

- autonomic dysfunction (55% incidence)
- sensory disturbance (50% incidence)
- weakness (75% incidence).

Autonomic dysfunction

Initially there is loss of bladder control, which progresses to retention and overflow incontinence.

Sweating does not occur below the level of the lesion.

Sensory disturbance

There is ascending loss of sensation with numbness which usually stops about one vertebral body below the level of the cord compression.

The patient may have a sensation of coldness.

Weakness

This usually starts as stiffness or unsteadiness and progresses to sensory disturbance.

Signs of compression

Look for the following:

- pain on neck flexing or straight leg raising
- pain or tenderness to percussion over the affected vertebrae
- palpable bladder with incomplete emptying
- sensory loss below the affected cord segment, with loss of pinprick, position and vibration senses
- sphincter tone is decreased on rectal examination.

Relevant investigations

The extent of investigations should be tailored to the condition and expected prognosis of the individual patient, and depends on what treatment can be tolerated.

Plain X-ray of the spine detects about 85% of spinal lesions, but a negative result does not exclude metastases. Lymphoma patients can have metastases without any findings on X-ray.

MRI scanning is more accurate, but is less comfortable for the patient because they have to lie still for much longer.

Myelography will determine the extent of the blockage and can be used if it is easier or faster than obtaining MRI scans.

℞ Remedy

Give dexamethasone 100 mg intravenously immediately, followed by a maintenance dose of between 16 and 96 mg per 24 hours in four divided doses.

Four types of treatment are available:

- chemotherapy
- radiotherapy
- steroids
- surgery.

Chemotherapy

Chemotherapy is indicated if there is a recurrence of responsive tumour following surgery or radiotherapy, or as adjuvant therapy in lymphomas and some other tumours. Prostate cancer may respond to hormone therapy without radiotherapy.

Radiotherapy

Radiation treatment can be used if there is no spinal instability and the tumour is known to be radiosensitive. It should be started immediately and may be given over 2 to 4 weeks.

The response depends on the tumour sensitivity, with lymphomas showing a good response, breast cancer a fair response and lung cancer a poor response.

Steroids

Steroids should be started immediately in all patients. In patients with a poor prognosis they are the only feasible treatment option. They have some anti-tumour action, reduce peri-tumour oedema, and may relieve pain and improve neurological function in the short term.

Having started with the dose quoted above, the dose should be reduced by one-third every 3 or 4 days and stopped after about 10 days, when there is either an improvement or it has been shown that the damage is irreversible.

Surgery

Surgery is an option in selected patients with a good prognosis. Indications for surgery include the following:

- failure to respond to irradiation
- radiation resistance
- relapse after successful irradiation
- spinal instability following pathological fracture.

E Extra information

Paraplegia due to malignant spinal cord compression is always irreversible and therefore is not an emergency as such.

Other causes of the symptoms suggestive of cord compression include the following:

- disc disease
- epidural abscess
- epidural haematoma.

Disc disease

This usually affects the lower lumbar vertebrae, and there is no mass on MRI scanning.

Epidural abscess

Fever is usually present and myelography should confirm the diagnosis.

Epidural haematoma

Patients usually have low platelet counts or are on anticoagulants. More than one vertebral segment is likely to be involved.

Further reading

- Eva G, Lord S. Rehabilitation in malignant spinal cord compression. *Eur J Palliat Care*. 2003; **10:** 148–50.
- Halkyard E. Recognising signs of malignant spinal cord compression. *Nurs Times*. 2004; **100:** 41.
- Joseph M, Tayar R. Spinal cord compression requires early detection. *Eur J Palliat Care*. 2005; **12:** 141–3.
- Purdue C. Diagnosis and treatment of malignant spinal cord compression. *Nurs Times*. 2004; **100:** 38–41.
- Shaw P, Marks A. Malignant spinal cord compression. *Eur J Palliat Care*. 2003; **10:** 141–4.

Chapter 46

Sweating

Obviously this method I have discovered is of great importance, since it enables us to ascertain the precise amount of that insensible perspiration interference which, according to Hippocrates and Galen, is the cause of all diseases.

Santorio Santorio (Italian physican and inventor of the clinical thermometer, 1561–1636)[1]

Introduction

Sweating is a normal physiological mechanism whereby the secretion of fluid on to the skin cools the body.

The severity of sweating is influenced by the environment, and what is regarded as 'normal' is very variable. There have been attempts to produce sweating severity scales, but none of these have been validated or tested for reliability.

About 5% of cancer patients experience troublesome sweating.

Night sweats are particularly associated with lymphomas and lung cancer.

C Consider

After excluding simple causes like a hot environment, the causes of sweating can be divided into two groups.

Common causes

- Disseminated malignancy, especially liver and kidney secondaries.
- Lymphomas.
- Sepsis (fever may be masked if the patient is on steroids).
- Sex hormone insufficiency (possibly associated with hormone therapies).

Less common causes

- Endocrine – for example, hypoglycaemia (which may be seen in diabetes mellitus as part of an autonomic neuropathy) or hypothyroidism.
- Fear and anxiety.
- Opioids.
- Pain.
- Reactions to blood, drugs, etc.
- Weakness.

A Assess

When did the attacks of sweating start? Is there any relationship to starting a new medication or the administration of a hormone-based treatment?

How severe are the attacks? Has the patient suffered from this problem before?

Check simple causes such as environmental conditions.

Look for signs of infection.
If indicated, check blood sugar levels and thyroid function.

℞ Remedy

General non-pharmacological measures

If a reversible cause has been identified, deal with this appropriately.

- Airflow should be increased by using a fan or opening a window.
- Cooler clothing (e.g. cotton), preferably quite loose fitting, should be worn.
- Humidity should be reduced.
- Temperature in the room should be adjusted.
- Tepid sponging should be undertaken frequently.

Sweating increases insensitive fluid loss. To counteract this, encourage a realistic fluid intake.

Pharmacological measures

Four main areas should be considered, namely infection, neoplastic fever, sex hormone insufficiency, and finally treatments that are non-specific, sometimes anecdotal rather than evidence based or pharmacologically explained, but effective.

Infection

- Acetaminophen (paracetamol) 1 g orally or rectally every 6 hours.
- Antibiotics if appropriate to the patient's general condition and prognosis. If an antibiotic will improve symptom control and general quality of life, it should be considered.

Neoplastic fever

- Naproxen, 250–500 mg twice daily orally helps about two-thirds of patients. Sometimes switching to a different NSAID (e.g. indometacin) helps. The mechanism for this is unclear.
- Steroids have been shown to help. The reason is unclear and there is no agreed starting dose, but it is common to try dexamethasone 2 mg in the morning and to adjust the dose to achieve an acceptable response.

Sex hormone insufficiency

- Clonidine 0.3–0.4 mg at night may help by stabilising blood vessel activity.
- Diethylstilboestrol 1–3 mg orally once daily may be helpful in *men*, but carries the risk of associated thromboembolic events.

Treatments worth trying

- Antimuscarinics (e.g. propantheline 15 mg orally at night) may help by blocking parasympathetic-mediated sweating.
- Beta-blockers.
- Cimetidine (particularly for opioid-induced sweating).
- Diltiazem.

How some of these treatments work is unclear, and the product licence may not support this use, but anecdotal accounts over several years consistently report that they are beneficial.

E Extra information

Disease involving the hypothalamus or pituitary gland (e.g. acromegaly) is a rare cause of sweating. Sometimes a rare 'hemibody' flushing and sweating is seen, where one side of the body is red and sweaty and the other side is normal.

Try, if possible, to choose an agent that simplifies the prescription (e.g. if the patient needs an NSAID, consider indometacin or naproxen depending upon the above considerations). If gastric protection is indicated, consider cimetidine.

Reference

1 Sigerist HE. *A Biographical History of Medicine.* New York: WW Norton and Co.; 1933.

Further reading

- Hami F, Trotman I. The management of sweating. *Eur J Palliat Care.* 1999; **6:** 184–7.

Chapter 47

Tenesmus

> As an adult she had her organs removed one by one. Now she is left with a mere shell, with symptoms where her organs used to be.
>
> William O Abbot (1902–1943)

Introduction

Tenesmus is an unpleasant sensation of rectal fullness and needing to open the bowels. It can occur after an abdomino-perineal resection of the rectum, in which case it is known as 'phantom rectum.'

Bladder tenesmus also occurs (*see* Extra information, p. 197).

C Consider

Tenesmus is due to pressure on the stretch receptors in the levator ani muscles.

It is usually caused by either a rectal tumour or pelvic recurrence. Impacted faeces can also cause the problem or make it worse.

What surgery or radiotherapy procedure has the patient undergone?

How long has the tenesmoid sensation been present and what has been offered to help? It is not uncommon for patients to be reluctant to admit to the symptom due to embarrassment and thinking that it sounds rather odd to report.

The pain felt in tenesmus often has nociceptive and neuropathic elements. Defaecation, even when 'successful', can cause worsening of the tenesmoid pain and is therefore associated with anxiety and fear.

A Assess

Exclude faecal impaction.

Is there a local tumour of the rectum? If so, is there any vaginal involvement in a female patient?

Is the tumour operable?

℞ Remedy

In many cases all that can be offered is symptom management, and no curative option is available. A number of options may be tried, with varying success. These include the following.

- Amitriptyline may help to block the nerve impulses that are being conducted.
- Anticonvulsants may reduce the number of unwanted nerve impulses and thus reduce the sensation.
- Bupivicaine enemas help some patients.
- Corticosteroids – high-dose steroids can reduce peri-tumour oedema and may ease the sensation of tenesmus.

- Glyceryl trinitrate (GTN) spray used on the anus, or 2% GTN ointment applied to the rectal mucosa, has been shown to be effective in tenesmus due to anal fissure (the products may not be licensed for this use).
- Laser therapy may be feasible for some tumours.
- Nifedipine in a modified-release formulation, 10–20 mg daily, may be used.
- NSAIDs may help.
- Opioids may help but are unreliable, as the pain is only partially opioid responsive.
- Radiotherapy can be helpful, but if there is vaginal involvement there is a risk of fistula formation.
- Rectal suppositories of NSAID or morphine may be helpful.
- Steroid enemas are sometimes helpful.

The number of options given reflects the fact that no single treatment is better than another.

E Extra information

Bilateral lumbar sympathetic nerve block can be considered if other measures have failed. The success rate is about 80%.

Spinal infusion of local anaesthetics, possibly with opioids added, is another possible option.

Bladder tenesmus causes the feeling of a full bladder and may be caused by a tumour enlarging either within the bladder or in the pelvis.

Bladder spasm and discomfort may also be associated with other bladder problems, including retention, infection, calculi, clots or even a catheter. These should be easily checked and dealt with.

Chapter 48

Terminal restlessness

> No one is moved to act or resolves to speak a single word, who does not hope by means of his action or word to release anxiety from his spirit.
>
> Ali ibn Hazm (Arab theologian, 994–1064) *To Apply to Souls*

Introduction

About 40% of terminally ill cancer patients become restless and agitated.

The underlying cause of restlessness may be physical, mental or a combination of both. It is therefore important to try to find out whether the patient can explain what is disturbing them.

C Consider

Ascertain whether the patient is showing any of the following behaviours:

- agitated – perhaps about some unfinished personal business
- anxious – about the treatment, the future, or dying
- confused – think about metabolic or biochemical causes
- moaning and groaning – think about pain
- semi-consciousness – could it be biochemical, or drug induced?
- tossing and turning – is the patient in pain or discomfort?

A Assess

Is the patient able to describe the problem or their fears?

Are those caring for the patient able to describe the problem, when it started and how it has developed?

Is the patient in any discomfort? Look for signs of the following:

- constipation
- dyspnoea
- full bladder
- itchy skin, with excoriation or scratch marks
- nausea
- pain.

Is the patient on any treatment or drugs that may be causing the restlessness? Think especially of steroids and neuroleptics.

℞ Remedy

Non-pharmacological measures

Adopt a reassuring approach and speak to the patient. If they are not alert, touch them as well, so that there are two sensory inputs to confirm your presence. Assume that they can hear and understand you.

Attempt to explain any underlying cause to the patient and their carers.

Reassure the patient and their carers about how you plan to deal with the situation.

Pharmacological measures

Chlorpromazine

Chlorpromazine is useful for terminal restlessness, and also helps pre-terminal dyspnoea. It can be given rectally, which is a useful property when used in the home situation. The usual dose is 25 mg per rectum up to four times daily.

Midazolam

A loading dose of 5 mg should be given subcutaneously, followed by 30 mg over 24 hours. More may be needed, up to a maximum dose of 60 mg in 24 hours.

Levomepromazine

Start with 25 mg over 24 hours and titrate according to response, up to 200 mg over 24 hours.

Phenobarbital

If all of the other regimes fail, start with 200 mg phenobarbital over 24 hours, increasing to a maximum of 600 mg if necessary.

Note: Phenobarbital cannot be used in combination with any other drug, and requires a second syringe driver.

E Extra information

If midazolam and levomepromazine are unavailable, promethazine, hyoscine hydrobromide or haloperidol are all suitable alternatives. It is important to note that promethazine and hyoscine can cause paradoxical agitation.

Cost is never the primary consideration when effective care is the aim, but it is interesting to note that the cost of midazolam is between 30 and 100 times that of chlorpromazine, depending on the doses required.

Further reading

- MacLeod S, Vella-Brincat J, Topp M. Terminal restlessness – is it a fair clinical concept? *Eur J Palliat Care*. 2004; **11:** 188–9.

Chapter 49

Twitching

Fasciculation: involuntary contractions or twitching of groups (fasciculi) of muscle fibres, a coarser form of muscular contraction than fibrillation.
Fascicle:
(1) A band or bundle of fibres, usually of muscle or nerve fibres; a nerve fibre tract.
(2) A section of a book that is published in instalments.

Introduction

Twitching is a non-specific term used to describe fine dyskinetic or abnormal involuntary movements. Tics, tremors and myoclonic jerks are included in the term 'twitching.'

Exclude the reversible causes of terminal restlessness before making this diagnosis.

Twitching should be distinguished from the normal fasciculations of wasted muscles.

C Consider

Are there any obvious metabolic abnormalities that are treatable?

Is the patient on any drugs that may be causative (e.g. phenothiazines, gastrokinetic agents or very-high-dose opioids)?

A Assess

Is the patient suffering from myoclonic jerks, tics or tremors?

Myoclonic jerks

Myoclonic jerks are rapid shock-like muscle jerks, which are often repetitive and sometimes rhythmic. Causes include the following:

- drugs
- metabolic causes
- myoclonic epilepsy
- opioids.

Drugs

Causative drugs are those that decrease the seizure threshold. The main ones are:

- antidopaminergic drugs
- butyrophenones
- domperidone
- metoclopramide

- phenothiazines
- tricyclic antidepressants.

Metabolic causes

Metabolic causes include the following:

- carbon dioxide narcosis
- hepatic failure
- hypercalcaemia
- hyponatraemia
- uraemia.

Opioids

Rarely, opioids may cause myoclonic jerks. This normally only occurs for two reasons:

1. the dose of opioid has been rapidly increased, *or*
2. the patient's previously normal renal function has deteriorated, resulting in an accumulation of the metabolic products of opioids.

Check renal function, and you may wish to check the serum levels of morphine metabolites to exclude morphine toxicity.

Tics

Tics are repetitive stereotyped movements that can be held in check voluntarily, but the concentration required exhausts and stresses the patient.

Tremors

A tremor is a rhythmic movement of a body part, caused by regular muscle contractions. Tremors can be of three types:

- intention tremor
- postural tremor
- resting tremor.

Intention tremors are seen in the following:

- brainstem disease
- cerebellar disease.

Postural tremor is a normal physiological variant, which may be exaggerated in the following:

- alcohol abuse
- anxiety
- thyrotoxicosis.

Resting tremor is seen in the following:

- extrapyramidal disease
- Parkinson's disease, including drug-induced Parkinsonism.

℞ Remedy

Discuss the causes with the conscious patient and with the relatives.

If possible, reduce the dose of any causative drug.

Treat any metabolic cause, such as hyponatraemia or hypercalcaemia.

If necessary, prescribe a benzodiazepine (e.g. diazepam or midazolam). Begin with a low dose and increase the dose until there is a response. The sedative effects of benzodiazepines will limit their use in conscious alert patients.

Review the patient daily.

E Extra information

In severely ill patients it is common to find combinations of all the causes listed above. For example, a patient on increasing doses of morphine for uncontrolled pain, who also requires an anti-emetic such as haloperidol, and who has an obstructive nephropathy from a large pelvic tumour has several reasons for developing twitching of their muscles.

Part 5

Practical issues in the care of the patient

Chapter 50

Discharge planning

> Discharges of patients from hospital have in the past been handled haphazardly by healthcare professionals. Coordination of this important part of a person's experience of hospital would have psychological and emotional benefits for patients, staff and the NHS as a whole.
>
> L Nazarko[1]

Introduction

Discharge planning takes time, and should therefore commence at the time of admission. On admission, information is gathered so that referrals to other members of the multi-disciplinary team can be made appropriately.

C Consider

The aims of discharge planning are as follows:

- to prepare the patient and their relatives for the patient's transfer home or to an agreed suitable environment for their effective and adequate care
- to facilitate smooth transfer of the patient without disruption to the care they require
- to promote, for as long as possible, as much independence as is realistic and to ensure that the care needed is within the abilities of the carers to provide
- to ensure continuity of appropriate care by effective and adequate communication between the discharging and receiving units.

The following information is required to achieve these aims.

Medical history

- What is the patient's main diagnosis?
- Does the patient have any other relevant medical conditions?
- What is their likely prognosis?
- Is there any sensory impairment that might prevent the patient from being self-caring?

Drug history

- Are all the current medications essential? Can the regime be simplified to ensure better compliance?
- How are the medications dispensed? Can the patient obtain his or her prescriptions?
- Can the patient self-medicate? If not, who is responsible for this?

Social and family history

- Who lives with the patient?
- What type of house does the patient live in? For example, are there stairs and can the patient manage these?
- Is access to the toilet easy for the patient to manage by him- or herself?
- Is the patient able to wash and dress independently?
- Who does the cooking?
- Who does the laundry?
- Who does the shopping?
- What services are already in place?
- Is any additional support required from other sources?

How well was the family coping prior to the patient's admission? What difficulties did it have?

Is anyone dependent on the patient for help? If so, how will they cope?

Is the primary care team happy to accept the patient back for care at home?

A Assess

The patient

Is the patient's disease progressing so that they require care in a place other than their own home? If so, where should this be? (*See* Chapter 51.)

If discharge home is considered possible, assess the patient's need for help with the following:

- activities of daily living
- cooking
- laundry
- shopping.

Is there a need for additional services that are not already in place?

The family

- How well was the family coping before this admission? Has there been a significant change in the patient's care requirements since admission?
- Is the family competent to take on the care that is now required?
- Is it confident about taking on the care required?
- Is it willing and prepared to take on the care required?

Is a home assessment required or a trial at home with the patient's bed kept for 48 hours in case home care is not feasible? While one appreciates the pressure on hospital and hospice beds, patients and their families are saved a lot of anxiety by knowing that there is a 'safety net' in case they cannot manage the care required. Honest, realistic discussion about the practical problems of caring at home can often alleviate or prevent guilt when the family tries its best but cannot manage the level of care that is needed.

Are there 'boundaries' or limits to what the family can do (e.g. bathing, assistance with using the toilet, etc.)? How are these going to be overcome? Ask about this specifically, and encourage the patient and relatives to be honest in their responses. This issue must be addressed and agreed before discharge, and one should not assume that either the patient or the family (including the patient's partner) finds this type of care acceptable.

The home

- Are any adaptations required? If so, are these needed before the patient is discharged? Who is responsible for seeing to this?

℞ Remedy

Throughout hospital admission it is essential to:

- involve all the appropriate therapy staff
- advise the discharge liaison staff, the GP and primary care team and the palliative care team of plans for discharge, so that all of the necessary arrangements are made before the patient comes home
- involve the patient and relatives in decisions about the date and place of discharge
- maintain the patient's independence
- make timely referrals to the social work department, recognising that it takes time for arrangements to be set up.

It is the role of the named nurse to coordinate the discharge plan. They have a responsibility to act as an advocate for the patient, to liaise with the multi-disciplinary team and to negotiate the best plan for the patient's care after discharge.

Look at the information gathered and the assessments made by therapy staff. Take into account any issues that may have arisen prior to admission and any change in the patient's condition since admission.

With this information to hand, have a discussion with the multi-disciplinary team to determine the best place for care to be offered. Explain the decision and the reasons for it to the patient and their relatives. Allow them to ask questions and express any anxieties they may have, and deal with these.

Explain to the patient and their family what to do if they are not coping with caring at home.

Agree an estimated or expected discharge date and inform all of the relevant agencies of this date as soon as possible to ensure that everything required is in place before discharge.

With regard to what is essential for discharge, consider each of the following:

- district nurse services to be organised
- equipment (e.g. raised toilet seat or commode)
- GP made aware of discharge and follow-up plans
- home help or home shopping services, etc.
- Macmillan nurse
- meals on wheels
- social worker
- other services specific to the patient's needs.

Who is to be contacted in an emergency? Make sure that the patient and relatives have all the relevant details and phone numbers.

Can adequate support and care be given at home or does consideration have to be given to alternative care, whether at a hospice or a care centre?

E Extra information

Not all discharges are successful. Some patients and their families desperately want to try at home, and they should be supported in doing so. Some will fail because the patient's condition deteriorates and is no longer compatible with care at home, but sadly some fail to cope due to inadequate planning. We can try to prevent these failures by:

- appropriate placement
- correct use of community services
- early involvement of all of the relevant agencies
- early preparation for discharge
- educational packages.

It has to be appreciated that some discharges will fail regardless of how well they are planned, generally because the patient's condition deteriorated in a way that could not be foreseen. This does not represent failure on the part of the family, and it should not feel guilty about not being able to continue to care for the patient at home.

Reference

1 Nazarko L. Improving discharge: the role of the discharge co-ordinator. *Nurs Standard.* 1998; **12:** 35–7.

Further reading

- Tarling M, Jauffur H. Improving team meetings to support discharge planning. *Nurs Times.* 2006; **102:** 32–5.
- Watson D. Planning to ensure the safe transfer of hospital patients. *Nurs Times.* 2006; **102:** 21–22.

Chapter 51

Where can the patient be cared for?

'She says, if you please, sir, she only wants to die in peace.'
'What! And the whole class to be disappointed? Impossible. Tell her she can't be allowed to die in peace; it is against the rules of the hospital!'

John F Murray (1811–1865), *The World of London*

Introduction

The majority of terminally ill people want to die at home. A poll taken in 2006 of people with long-term health conditions and disabilities showed that this was the wish of 90% of the respondents. Unfortunately, only a few have their wish granted. While planning their care it sometimes becomes apparent that it hasn't been thought through or adequately discussed and, as a result, adequate preparations were not made in time.

Wherever end-of-life care is provided it is essential that everyone involved is open and honest with the patient. The patient may want to be cared for at home but fails to appreciate the practical difficulties or the time required to set up the services necessary to fulfil this request.

The options are as follows:

- hospital
- hospice
- care centres
- home.

Because home care requires the most planning, it will be discussed in the greatest detail.

Hospital

Acute settings are not ideal. They are very busy and often lack single rooms where people can spend time in privacy with their family and friends. The focus is not solely on palliative care, and acutely ill patients take priority.

If a patient is admitted as an emergency, notes from previous admissions are often difficult to access immediately, and therefore inappropriate treatments may be given.

Hospice

The strength of the hospices is their focus on symptom control and their expertise in this area. Beds are not always readily available, and most hospices have a demand for beds that makes it difficult for them to offer medium- to long-stay care. The hospices do provide day care and home care services.

Day care is now a major part of the hospice service. Depending on the patient's fitness, arrangements may be made for attendance once or more each week. This allows the relatives to have time for other duties and activities.

Day care units or centres offer respite for the carer and provide peer-group support for the patient. A wide range of creative and social activities is provided, as well as nursing and medical input, physiotherapy, occupational therapy, complementary therapies, hairdressing, chiropody and beauty treatments.

Care centres

Care centres are less busy than acute settings, and more priority is given to palliative care. Residents have their own rooms, thus allowing private time with family and friends.

On admission, care plans are formulated and discussions about care are documented.

Care is provided by registered nurses and carers, working together with GPs and family members.

As part of the NHS End of Life Programme, the Department of Health and the National Council for Palliative Care published an introductory guide for care homes in May 2006. This is the first of a planned series of publications. Visit the website www.endoflifecare.nhs.uk for further details, as this is a developing programme.

Home

Provision of care at home is what most patients would like, but many do not receive it. Since it is the most challenging option, it will be dealt with in more detail.

C Consider

While for most people care at home is the desired option, it can be difficult to facilitate. A great deal of thought has to be given to who will provide the care. Services in the community are usually very busy, and often family members and friends are the care providers. This puts pressure on family and friends, and encroaches on their 'quality time'. It can be very tiring and stressful, partly because the family needs to be available 'round the clock'. Any difficulties or crises often result in hospital admission.

When the patient asks to go home for a few days, this is probably because he or she wants to:

- see home for the last time
- be with the family and be 'in control', even for a very short time
- complete some unfinished (private) business
- reflect on his or her situation and get the illness into perspective.

It can be helpful for the family to be involved in the care of the patient. The patient needs their presence and support. The relatives need to feel involved, and they want to alleviate the effects of the disease on their loved one. This is most often expressed in a wish to provide some practical help for the patient. It would be a disservice to the relative if they were left with a belief that they had 'failed' in caring for the patient.

A Assess

When the appropriate place is identified, it is important to identify what if any reasons would necessitate the patient being moved from there, and to put measures in place to ensure that those circumstances do not arise. Careful and precise care planning is essential.

- What are the patient's specific needs?
- In which setting can they be best met?
- Can they be met at home for some of the time?

Establish the following facts from the relatives.

- Who is available to help?
- What kind of help are they able to offer?
- As a family, can they realistically provide help day and night?

It is not uncommon for families to make an offer of help that is genuinely meant, but unrealistic and impossible to provide. If they have not been in this situation before, they probably do not realise the workload they are offering to take on.

Find out whether the care that the relatives can comfortably provide is limited to, for example, helping to provide drinks and food or assisting the patient with eating. Limited help is not unimportant help, but it must be established who is responsible for more intimate care, such as helping to wash the patient. Some relatives may find these tasks extremely difficult.

It is important not to assume that a patient and relative (including the patient's partner) have had an intimate relationship in the past. Always find out what is acceptable to the patient and the carer.

Ask the patient what their own wishes and expectations are.

- Who can offer support at home? Is there a partner, a son or daughter, a parent, a relative, a friend, or no one?
- What general ability (physical and mental) does each carer have?
- Does anyone have any experience as a carer, a nurse or in any other area of healthcare provision?
- What is the age of the carer(s)? Can they be expected to cope?
- For how much of the day and night is the home carer available?
- What is the carer's perspective on the aims of care?
- What is the home like? Think about things like stairs, access to a toilet, availability of a telephone, cooking facilities and the general needs of the patient, and how well these needs are matched by the facilities at home.

℞ Remedy

Following discussions with the multi-professional team members, plan a strategy for involving relatives in the care of the patient. Include as many of the normal activities of daily living as possible (e.g. washing, dressing, meal provision).

Discuss with both the patient and the family how well they coped and whether they feel confident that they can manage at home.

Make sure that they are aware that no guarantee can be given that a hospital or hospice bed will always be readily available locally, and discuss how they would be able to care for the patient if he or she deteriorated suddenly or lost consciousness in the terminal stage.

The GP must be in agreement with the decision that the patient should be cared for at home, and should be aware of the input that the specialist palliative care team can offer.

When planning the discharge home, contact the GP and the district nurse in order to:

- enquire about what community support is available
- discuss the patient's physical abilities/needs and treatment regimes (e.g. syringe driver)
- inform them of the patient's and the family's understanding of the disease and the prognosis
- discuss the input needed from the Macmillan nurse or palliative care team
- confirm that the patient has an adequate supply of medication on discharge
- discuss a possible need for readmission with the GP.

It is important to confirm these arrangements in writing when the patient is discharged. This ensures that deputising staff can be informed what arrangements have been agreed.

Meet with the patient and carers in order to:

- inform them of the support available at home
- inform them of your communication with the GP and support team, and tell the family carers who each person is and what they do
- discuss with them what to do if things go wrong, and whom to contact – a written list of contact names and phone numbers is invaluable
- check that they understand the drug regime, which should be in writing.

If possible, keep the bed available for 1 or 2 days in case there is a need for an early return to hospital. This is the ideal, but the patient and their carers must be aware that the 'real-world' situation is that another patient may require the bed urgently.

Some localities now have home respite teams who will provide up to 24-hour home nursing care in the last few days of life. As well as facilitating discharge home to die, these services can obviate the need for 'last-minute' admission to a hospital or hospice.

E Extra information

Returning home, even for a few days, enhances the patient's autonomy and therefore their self-esteem.

If the patient is moving from an acute setting, good discharge planning is essential. As well as looking at personal activities of daily living, thought should be given to the following:

- district nurse/carer input required
- equipment required
- meal provision
- administration of medication
- overnight arrangements.

Failed discharges are usually the result of poor planning. It has often been said that discharge planning should commence on admission.

The 'negative' aspects of care at home are as follows.

- There is pressure on the family.
- 'Quality time' is limited due to the workload of care provision.

- There is no 24-hour nursing input as such. The family provides 24-hour care with visits from the nurse.
- Carer input increases dramatically in the terminal phase. The family should be aware of this and should be helped with planning for this time.
- Options for crisis management at home are limited, and this often results in hospital admission.

Carers should be reassured that some help and support is available for the patient and the family at home. Usually it is arranged prior to discharge through the GP, the care manager from social services and community nursing staff. Be aware that it can take a few days for services to be fully set up, and equipment loan and delivery can also take a few days, so plan in advance and be aware of public holidays and other reasons for delays or reduced service provision. Remind the patient that they should return any equipment quickly when it is no longer required, as a delay in returning equipment results in a delay in someone else getting it on loan.

Prior to discharge, the patient and their relatives should be shown simple methods of lifting the patient or helping him or her to transfer from bed to chair. They should be competent and confident in doing this before the patient is discharged.

Help and support at home also includes aids such as a bath seat, a wheelchair, a commode, a handrail to ease climbing stairs, or blocks to raise the height of a chair or bed. These may make an enormous difference to a patient's independence. Check which service provides these aids in your area and how they are returned when they are no longer needed.

Other services available to help with care at home are summarised below.

Community care

Social services have a statutory responsibility under community care legislation to conduct community care assessments that take account of the needs of individuals and also the needs of their carers. Since April 1966 the Carers (Recognition and Services) Act allows carers to have a separate assessment of their needs, should they wish it.

To avoid inappropriate delays in the date of discharge, early referral to the social worker is essential to ensure that the assessment process is undertaken as early as possible.

Remember that the GP will be in charge of the patient's care at home. To facilitate good care, they must be fully informed of plans to discharge the patient and given adequate time to ensure that all necessary support is available.

Community nursing

District nurses can provide practical nursing help with dressings, supervision of medication, bathing and other nursing tasks.

Day care units

Day care units that offer a large range of services are now widely available.

Equipment for patient care

A variety of physical aids may be obtained following assessment by the occupational therapist, who can then order any equipment that will be necessary.

Financial support

It is advisable to consult a social worker to check for recent changes and amendments to welfare benefits, but Disability Living Allowance or Attendance Allowance may be payable.

Macmillan grants may be made for any reasonable and practical necessity. Further information is available from their website at www.macmillan.org.uk.

Patients with a progressive illness who are not reasonably expected to live for more than 6 months can apply for Disability Living Allowance and Attendance Allowance under the Special Rules. From September 2006 these grants are payable for a fixed period of 3 years, and a renewal claim form will be sent to the claimant 6 months before the award is due to expire. Further information is available from the website of the Department for Work and Pensions at www.dwp.gov.uk.

There are various benevolent societies, particularly for ex-servicemen, retired actors and actresses and other groups. One of these may provide financial support for a suitable patient. Most patients who are eligible for such support will know how to contact the relevant bodies.

Meals-on-wheels service

This service, which is normally provided by local authorities, delivers a hot midday meal daily to the home, and may be the mainstay of the patient's diet. A nominal charge is made.

Practical help in the home

Practical aid may be provided by a home help, who is employed by the local authority. Referral is via the local social services department.

Marie Curie nurses may be available to provide night-time or 24-hour home care.

Private practical or nursing help

Commercial agencies in most areas will put relatives and patients in touch with domestic help, companions or nurses.

Further reading

- Borgsteede SD, Graafland-Riedstra C, Deliens L *et al.* Good end-of-life care according to patients and their GPs. *Br J Gen Pract.* 2006; **56:** 20–26.
- Collins F. An evaluation of palliative care services in the community. *Nurs Times.* 2004; **100:** 34–7.
- Deschepper R, Vander Stichele R, Bernheim JL *et al.* Communication on end-of-life decisions with patients wishing to die at home. *Br J Gen Pract.* 2006; **56:** 14–19.

- Edwards A, Hirst P. Supporting palliative care in care homes – the way forward? *Eur J Palliat Care.* 2005; **12:** 64–8.
- Ewing G, Rogers M, Barclay S *et al.* Palliative care in primary care. *Br J Gen Pract.* 2006; **56:** 27–34.
- Gomes B, Higginson I. Home or hospital? Choices at the end of life. *J R Soc Med.* 2004; **97:** 413–14.
- Matthews K, Finch J. Provision of palliative care education in nursing homes. *Nurs Times.* 2006; **102:** 36–40.
- Matthews K, Finch J. Using the Liverpool Care Pathway in a nursing home. *Nurs Times.* 2006; **102:** 34–5.
- Payne S, Kerr C, Hawker S *et al.* Community hospitals: an under-recognized resource for palliative care. *J R Soc Med.* 2004; **97:** 428–31.
- Worth A, Boyd K, Kendall M *et al.* Out-of-hours palliative care: a qualitative study of cancer patients, carers and professionals. *Br J Gen Pract.* 2006; **56:** 6–13.

Chapter 52

The family as carers

> The physician that bringeth love and charity to the sick, if he be good and kind and learned and skilful, none can be better than he.
>
> Girolamo Savonarola (Italian religious and political reformer, 1452–1498) (Attrib.)

Introduction

It can be very helpful for a family to be involved in the care of the patient. The patient needs their presence and support and, for many relatives, helping to care for their dying loved one is a way of expressing their commitment and being satisfied that they could have done no more. This may help them to cope during bereavement.

Family members almost always need to feel that they are being helpful in some way. This is most often expressed in a desire to be able to offer practical help to the patient. If at all possible, try to accommodate this wish whilst ensuring that a 'safety net' is in place to support the family and see that they are not overwhelmed by the responsibilities involved in providing care. The last thing one wants is for a family to be left with a belief that they have 'failed' in their attempts to care for the patient.

C Consider

A relative's wish to be more involved may simply reflect the fact that they feel that they are not receiving sufficient information about the patient's illness and progress. They may think that by taking the patient home they will become more aware of what is really happening.

Who wishes to provide this help? Is it the relatives, or is the patient wishing to go home and putting pressure on the family to comply with this desire?

Does the patient share the relatives' desire that he or she should go home or stay at home?

In what way does the family wish to become more involved?

Could this be due to the relatives attempting to deal with their own needs, or their guilt about being seen as unable to cope?

Is adequate support available in the community to make home care feasible?

Is it possible that, by satisfying the wishes of the relatives, there could be a disruption to treatment that might have benefited the patient, or that his or her care might be compromised in some way?

A Assess

Find out what kind of help the family wishes to offer, and assess their ability to help. Care at home is a 'round-the-clock' commitment. Can they realistically provide this care?

Sometimes fears about caring at home are realistic, but sometimes the relatives are worrying about things that will never happen. How realistic are the hopes, fears and expectations that they have expressed?

The care that a relative can realistically offer may vary considerably. Some can only offer limited care, such as helping to provide drinks and food or helping the patient to eat. Care that is limited to simple input of this type is not unimportant, and should be encouraged.

What help is required now? Find out whether there is currently any input, or the need for input, from any of the following people:

- clinical nurse specialist
- district nurse
- domiciliary care (home help, meals on wheels)
- family doctor
- hospice day care
- Macmillan nurse
- social worker.

There are many others you may think of as well.

Has the GP been made aware of the patient's current situation and needs and any plans for this short-term or long-term discharge? He or she might have very valuable knowledge of the home circumstances that could influence your decision.

A Macmillan grant may help to provide an essential piece of equipment (e.g. washing machine, food liquidiser), enabling the family to cope better.

The patient may require more intimate care, such as help with bathing or washing. Some relatives may find these tasks extremely difficult. It is important not to assume that a patient and their relative have had an intimate relationship in the past. Always find out what is acceptable to the patient and the carer, including the patient and their partner.

Caring for a patient at home is often the cause of a great deal of stress. Before agreeing that the family is ready to take on the care of the patient, think about the following issues.

- What is the duration of the patient's illness and the stage of their illness?
- Has new information been shared that has prompted this request for home care? Has a new treatment begun that has resulted in some improvement?
- Has the patient's condition deteriorated and do the family want to be together while they think that this is still possible?
- What are the relationships within the family?
- How dependent is the patient on his or her relatives? Can they realistically cope?
- Are other demands being made on the relatives?
- What are the financial pressures as a result of the illness? Will caring at home result in loss of income through inability to attend work?

To avoid becoming over-stressed and unable to cope, the family needs the following:

- adequate support at home with the patient
- encouragement to deal with their own health problems, both physical and psychological

- help with meeting and talking as a family about their concerns
- help with exploring their own feelings
- regular rest and time to relax – not just to give care day and night, 7 days a week
- to be aware of any changes in treatment
- your 'permission' to have some time for themselves.

℞ Remedy

It has been said that 'to fail to plan is to plan to fail'. Planning and anticipation of problems are very important when setting up a suitable package for care at home.

Plan, with the multi-professional team members, a strategy for involving relatives in care where feasible (e.g. meal preparation, shaving, bathing), and encourage the relatives to assist in nursing the patient while he or she is in the hospital or hospice. This will help them to learn new skills, and it also allows the staff to assess these and, if necessary, to teach new techniques.

Discuss with the team members how competent the relatives have been in caring, and try to address any problems that might arise.

Explore the feelings of the relatives and deal with any issues that they raise with regard to their abilities and their perceived needs, both in terms of the patient and in relation to themselves as carers.

Allow participation with the patient's care and encourage the relatives to continue, as they feel able, to be involved in the care of the patient who loses consciousness in the terminal stage, thus making home care impossible.

In order to provide effective patient care at home you will need to establish detailed contact with the carers and with local support services. The occupational therapist can help by allowing the patient and the relatives to explore the practicalities. This can be achieved by carrying out a pre-discharge home assessment visit with the patient if he or she is able. If not, the occupational therapist can visit the house to look at the layout and offer advice to the carers with regard to what level of assistance is needed and any adaptations that are required for good patient care. Adaptations can take time, and the relatives need to be aware that patients sometimes deteriorate suddenly and that care at home may not be possible after all.

Some patients who are being cared for at home may be suitable for attendance at a day care unit. This allows the relatives to have time for other duties and activities, keeps the patient in touch with the hospital or hospice staff, and offers the patient a wide range of creative and social activities, as well as medical input, physiotherapy, occupational therapy, hairdressing, chiropody and beauty treatments.

It can be difficult to decide whether a patient should go home or stay at home. Some localities now have home respite teams that provide home nursing care for substantial portions of the day and night during the last few days of life. As well as facilitating discharge of the patient to die at home, if this is what the patient and the family want, this input may mean that admission to a hospital or hospice at the end of the illness can be avoided.

Before arranging transfer home, it is a good policy to check what services exist in your area and to discuss the appropriateness of the available services with the patient and their family as the carers.

It is advisable to explore with the patient's GP what support will be available when the patient is discharged. Discussing this well in advance of a planned discharge date allows adequate time for all the necessary services to be organised.

Despite good planning, unforeseen problems can develop rapidly and the patient's needs and condition can change suddenly, necessitating an urgent re-admission.

Admission for end-of-life care may leave carers feeling that they have failed, especially if they have made promises to allow the relative to die at home.

Advise relatives that it is always safest to make *plans*, not *promises*!

E Extra information

Offering all the available and appropriate support to the relatives will lead to better supported patients. It is essential to consider the social context in which patients and relatives are conducting their lives as they face death. The patient and their family should be offered the services of the social worker, nursing staff and all other agencies that are relevant to their needs.

The possibility of respite should be included in discussions and plans for future care at home.

Explore the relatives' existing coping strategies and help to develop them. You may well see a considerable difference in a family that has been able to discuss its problems openly and without fear of being seen as 'failing' when the burden of care becomes too great.

It is important to appreciate the effects of the stress that a family experiences while watching the disease progress. Family members who have been distressed from a very early point in the treatment process might well be exhausted by the time the patient enters the palliative phase of treatment. These families cannot be blamed for finding it hard to cope.

Sometimes the family wants to care for the patient at home because they are finding it difficult to cope with the cost of visiting the hospital. The Department of Health has published guidance on this subject in the document *The Hospital Travel Costs Scheme*. (A copy of this can be obtained by phoning 08701 555455, and it can also be downloaded by visiting www.doh.gov.uk/hospitaltravelcosts/hospitaltravelcostguidance.pdf)

The booklet *Caring for Someone Who is Dying* is one of the Carers' Handbooks published by Age Concern. (This useful resource can be obtained from Age Concern Books, Units 5 and 6, Industrial Estate, Brecon, Powys LD3 8LA. Tel: 0870 442 2120.)

Help the Aged also produces a series of booklets, including *Planning for the End of Life*, *Planning for Choice in End-of-Life Care* and *Listening to Older People*. These guides include discussion about caring, coping, ethical and legal issues and spirituality. (To obtain copies, contact Help the Aged, 207–221 Pentonville Road, London N1 9UZ. Tel: 020 7278 1114. Email: publications@help the aged.org.uk or download them from their website www.helptheaged.org.uk).

Further reading

- HM Government. *Palliative Care. Fourth Report of Session, 2004;* www.parliament.uk/parliamentarycommittees/health_committee.cfm
- Looi YC. For better or worse – till death do us part. *Geriatr Med*. 2006; **36:** 19–22.
- Mourman V. End-of-life patient-controlled analgesia at home. *Eur J Palliat Care*. 2005; **12:** 18–21.
- Nicholas S. Caring for carers: GPs in new charity collaboration. *New Generalist*. 2006; **4:** 55.

Chapter 53

The patient is dying

When a man lies dying, he does not die from the disease alone. He dies from his whole life.

Charles Péguy (1873–1914), *Basic Verities*

Introduction

Many families will have some prior experience of death either as individuals or as a group. These experiences may colour their expectations and prompt specific anxieties and fears depending on whether they have good or bad memories of the previous death.

The family may be seeking advice, comfort, company and regular visits for reassurance, or they may wish to be alone during those last few days or hours.

As the patient approaches death, he or she is making an unfamiliar journey. The family often has no clear idea of what may happen or what role to play. They may wish to discuss certain practical issues such as death certificates and registration, cremation, funeral plans, etc. Some patients wish to be involved and plan their own funeral, while others do not wish to address the issue in any way. Sensitivity is required.

It is important for the professional carers to agree that the patient is dying and for appropriate end-of-life care to be planned. Reversible possibilities such as hypercalcaemia should be considered. Agreement should be reached about whether to treat infections. The appropriate prognostic indicators such as rising urea and creatinine levels and low serum albumin levels should be monitored if necessary and appropriate, but it is inappropriate to carry out investigations if no action will be taken. When the team is agreed that death is inevitable, the end-of-life care package that is normally used by the team should be implemented.[1]

C Consider

The patient and their family are probably thinking about several things, including the following:

- changes in the patient's condition – what will happen and when?
- death – what will it be like to die?

The family may be asking themselves the following questions.

- Should we be here all the time? Is it permissible to take a short break?
- Should we be present at the moment of death? Some people wish to be present, others do not wish to, but may feel obliged to be present.
- Should we talk to the patient or touch the patient – before and after the death?
- Should we discuss our feelings and concerns with the patient?
- When and how do we say 'goodbye'?

The question of whether to be there all the time is a difficult one. Families may sit by the bedside for hours or days and the death can occur when they take a short break for a meal. This can lead to inappropriate guilt if they are not present at the moment of death, even if they have been there 'round the clock'. It is important for them to recognise the loving, caring input that they have given, and they should be helped to deal with their understandable anxiety and emotions related to not being present at the moment of death.

A Assess

How are the relatives feeling? Look for verbal and non-verbal cues.

Are there any questions that need to be answered?

Assess how much they want to be involved in caring for the patient.

Are they aware of the fact that the patient's death is quite imminent? Do they need to inform other family members, possibly sending for close relatives who live at a distance? Relatives who live some distance away may be less aware of the fact that the patient's condition could change suddenly. Avoidable delays can result in guilt about failing to 'get there in time'. Be realistic – don't let relatives risk having an accident by trying to make a hasty journey to see the patient before he or she dies if this is very unlikely or impossible. Sometimes, even with the best planning and predictions, patients deteriorate suddenly and die before their relatives can see them. It is always best to make contact with more distant relatives early on to allow more time for travelling.

How are the relatives coping with the stress of the situation?

Are there any particular religious or cultural practices that need to be observed before and after the death? The family may raise the issue, but it is best to find out rather than to let it be assumed that you knew about these.

℞ Remedy

Make sure that you are accessible as the death approaches, and make every effort to ensure continuity of care.

Sitting with a dying person can be very stressful and, if possible, all of the team members should try to evaluate the tension and stress within the family during this time.

Keep the patient and the family informed of the changing situation. Your regular visits will reduce tension within the family. If your visits coincide with visits by other members of the team, this gives everyone an opportunity to communicate, and it reinforces the team approach to the care of the patient and the availability of the whole team for the support of the patient and their family.

Encourage the relatives to disengage themselves temporarily from the caring situation. Breaks in continuity should be anticipated and a changeover period of shared care arranged. Often both the relatives and the patient need to realise that other carers are competent, and that in the event of any change in the patient's condition the relatives will be informed immediately.

Encourage the relatives to be involved, and let them know that their efforts are valued and that they are doing the right things.

The death may occur when a family member is taking a short break. Help that person not to feel guilty about this, by focusing on the amount of input that they gave throughout the illness.

Constant reassurance is required. In highly charged emotional situations like this, how one absorbs, understands and retains information is often far from perfect. Explanation of the situation may need to be repeated. Death is often peaceful, and this fact may need to be emphasised and the family reassured about this.

Provide guidance for those who find it difficult to relate to a dying person. Some families seem to know instinctively how to handle death. Others need encouragement to touch and talk to a dying relative. Relatives usually handle their loss better if they are present at the moment of death, and better still if a member of the team is also present. Reassure them that it is right to touch or kiss the dead person if they wish to do so. Equally, if any member of the family does not wish to be present when the death occurs, this is their right and they must do whatever they feel comfortable doing.

If they so wish, leave the family alone for a short time of private grief with the patient. Some will want this, and some will not. What is 'right' is what they feel comfortable with.

E Extra information

When patients are being cared for at home, it is helpful and reassuring to provide the family with the telephone numbers of all available members of the team involved in the patient's care. One often fears that such availability may encourage excessive dependence on the professional, but most families cope well and only call if they have good reasons for doing so.

After the death, consider the following.

- Did the patient die peacefully?
- Who was present at the time of death?

Invite the relatives to comment on anything that was not done as they hoped, and consider any lessons you might have learned from the management of this patient.

Did the organisation of the multi-professional team stand up to the pressure of managing a dying patient? Could it have been done better? If so, plan a meeting to deal with any areas that need improvement.

Are there any signs that the relatives will not be able to cope with their bereavement? What do you need to address in this context?

References

1 Campbell S. *Exploring Nursing and Medical Decision-making at the End of Life in Palliative Care Within the Hospital Setting.* MSc dissertation, Queen Margaret University College, Edinburgh, 2006.

Further reading

- Field D, Wee B. Preparation for palliative care: teaching about death, dying and bereavement in UK medical schools, 2000–2001. *Med Educ.* 2002; **36:** 561–7.

- Neuberger J. *Caring for Dying People of Different Faiths.* Oxford: Radcliffe Publishing; 2004.
- Neuberger J. *Dying Well: a guide to enabling a good death.* Oxford: Radcliffe Publishing; 2004.
- Somerville E, Mahyoub M, Hales K *et al.* Adapting the Liverpool Care Pathway for the dying patient. *Eur J Palliat Care.* 2005; **12:** 239–42.
- Stevenson J, Abernethy AP, Miller C *et al.* Managing comorbidities at the end of life. *BMJ.* 2004; **329:** 909–12.
- Taylor A. Improving practice with the Liverpool Care Pathway. *Nurs Times.* 2005; **101:** 36–7.

Chapter 54

Speaking to the relatives after a death

A man's dying is more the survivors' affair than his own.
Thomas Mann (1875–1955), *The Magic Mountain*

Introduction

Before you speak to the relatives, assuming that you were not present at the time of death, it is always helpful to know some basic facts.

- What was the nature of the death?
- Were the relatives present?
- What were the relationships between the patient and the family members? Is there any 'unresolved business' that needs to be addressed?
- Do other people need to be there (e.g. other family or team members who had a particularly close relationship with the patient)?

C Consider

However peaceful and expected it may be, death is a painful experience for relatives. It might be necessary to hear the expression of negative feelings at this time. Often, because of stress, events may not be seen in their true perspective. This is an opportunity to clarify any uncertainties and deal with any misunderstandings. It may be helpful to invite the relatives to ask about anything they did not understand and to express any concerns they had about the care that was given. Address genuine complaints – many of the comments will probably only need simple explanation or clarification. By addressing these, you may help to ease the pain of the loss and bereavement.

Think about how the relatives are feeling, and be sensitive in your approach.

Be aware of previous 'danger signals' which indicate that relatives might find it difficult to cope with the loss. These include the following:

- denial by the patient and/or relatives of the seriousness of the illness
- disputes and disagreements between the patient and their family
- recent bereavement.

What may the family wish to say to you? Consider offering extra support and possibly referring the family to the social worker at an early stage.

A Assess

Think about what the family might want to do now. They might wish to:

- contact other relatives who may come to the hospital for support or to take them home
- go home and return later for the death certificate and the patient's personal belongings

- see the patient again and spend some time with their loved one – they may wish to see the patient alone or with you
- sort out the patient's belongings in order to avoid having to make a second visit to collect these.

Be prepared for a variety of wishes to be expressed, and be ready to try to accommodate these as far as is possible in a busy ward with other patients watching.

Think about the privacy that is needed by the family at this time.

If concerns have been raised about any aspect of the patient's care, what action do you need to take?

℞ Remedy

Confirm that death has occurred. After sitting watching an immobile patient who is hardly breathing, the family may be unsure if the death has actually happened. While it may be appropriate to use gentle words at first, one must also use words like 'is dead' or 'has died' to reinforce that this final event has occurred.

Express your own feelings simply with expressions like 'I am very sorry.'

There is no single right way to respond to relatives when the patient has died. You will probably have already developed a relationship with both the patient and the family. You may well be feeling sad yourself.

Acknowledge the input that the relatives have given. Some will have wanted more practical involvement than others, but acknowledgement of their presence with the patient and recognition of the stressful time that they are going through is always appreciated.

Give the relatives the opportunity and time to ask you questions in order to aid their understanding of the situation. Give clear but caring responses.

Show the relatives the death certificate, confirming the patient's details and explaining any medical terms used, as these often cause confusion and anxiety later as the relatives sit wondering what the unfamiliar words actually mean.

There are practical issues to consider when a patient dies. It will help the relatives if you can provide information about the following:

- collecting the death certificate and registering the death
- cremation or burial, and the need for a second doctor to see the body and for extra forms to be completed for cremation. If the death occurred at home and a second doctor wishes to call to see the body before removal to the chapel of rest, this should be explained. Some families are concerned that they are under some kind of suspicion, and these fears must be dealt with
- follow-up and care during the time of bereavement
- funeral planning and the role of the undertaker
- reasons for carrying out a post-mortem.

Explain how to arrange the funeral. Most undertakers will offer a very comprehensive service, but sometimes the family have specific requests or wishes that they need to explore.

Discuss with the family what difficulties they anticipate, how they think they will handle them and whether they would like professional help. Offer practical help from yourself or the wider team as appropriate.

Make sure that you contact others who need to know that the death has occurred. This should be done promptly.

- Contact the patient's GP as soon as possible if death has occurred in a hospital or hospice. Leave a telephone message initially to ensure that the GP is aware of the death, and follow this up with a letter without undue delay. If this is relevant, comment on how the relatives are currently coping with their loss. Failure to do so can cause much avoidable stress and embarrassment.
- Contact all of the hospital consultants and clinics involved to cancel any arranged follow-up appointments if the death occurred in the community.

E Extra information

Leaflet D49, *What to Do After a Death*, is available from local Benefits Agency offices or by post from the Benefits Agency Storage and Distribution Centre, Manchester Road, Heywood, Lancashire OL10 2PZ. Most hospitals keep supplies to give to relatives with the death certificate.

In Scotland, the booklet *What to Do After a Death in Scotland* is available from DSS offices and is usually stocked by hospitals and hospices.

Sometimes it is necessary to report the death to the coroner (or the Procurator Fiscal in Scotland).

This usually causes anxiety to the relatives. You should acknowledge this anxiety and explain that there is no suspicion directed at their care. Some of the circumstances in which deaths must be reported are listed below. The full list is contained within the book of medical certificates for recording cause of death.

- Cause of death unknown.
- Deaths not due to natural causes, or where suicide or other suspicious action may be a factor.
- Deaths suspected of being related to drugs.
- Deaths occurring within 24 hours of an operation or an anaesthetic.
- Deaths occurring within 24 hours of admission to hospital.
- Deaths related to industrial disease – even if the latter is only a contributory factor, and if the patient was receiving an Industrial Injury or Disability Pension related to the cause of death.
- Deaths related to or alleged to be related in any way to injury.
- Cases where the doctor (usually the GP) has not seen the patient for 14 days prior to death.
- Cases where there has been any mishap, or where there has been criticism of nursing or medical care.

In addition, although very few patients in a palliative care setting are likely to be organ donors (with the possible exception of corneas), all deaths of potential organ donors must be reported to the Coroner.

Explain the legal obligations and the reason for reporting the death to the Coroner to the relatives. It is essential to explain to the relatives that reporting the death to the Coroner does not mean an automatic post-mortem examination or inquest, nor does it imply an automatic delay in arranging the funeral.

In some areas of Wales, *all* deaths of ex-miners must be reported routinely to the Coroner.

Further reading

- Lomas C. Gaining consent for post-mortems. *Nurs Times.* 2006; **102:** 58–9.
- Teasdale K. Care of the bereaved when postmortems are required. *Nurs Times.* 2004; **100:** 32–3.
- Weller S. *The Daily Telegraph Guide to Funerals and Bereavement.* London: Kogan Page; 1999.

Chapter 55

Bereavement

> To the atheist, death is the end; to the believer, the beginning; and to the agnostic, the sound of silence.
>
> Laurence Peter

Introduction

People vary in how they cope with bereavement. It is worth trying to assess which of the carers appears to be in greatest need of counselling. In particular, the needs of younger relatives and children in the family must not be overlooked.

C Consider

After the death the family may want time to clarify various issues with regard to the patient's illness and its management. These are usually simple, but misunderstandings can make bereavement and the grieving process more complicated.

If you work in the community, being accessible to the bereaved usually involves making special visits to the principal carers. These can be time-consuming, but are very helpful to the bereaved relatives.

A Assess

How are the relatives coping? Would the patient's partner or close relative benefit from referral to a support agency such as CRUSE?

Is professional counselling required by any of the relatives?

℞ Remedy

Visit the principal carers as soon as possible after the death. Other members of the team may also wish to visit after the death, and should be encouraged to do so.

In the community, it helps if the team coordinates their visits so that they visit at different times rather than on the same day! Gradually the time between visits can be elongated as the family copes with its loss.

Seeing the family at about 3 and 6 weeks after the death helps the family and facilitates their recovery.

Relatives often welcome a frank discussion with members of the team on how they felt about the deceased person and the management of the case. It also helps relatives to openly discuss their feelings.

All members of the team should try to evaluate whether the relatives are coping with their grief. Recognising the deterioration in physical health that occurs in many widows and widowers, advice on general health may well be appropriate.

E Extra information

Be aware of religious rites when you are interacting with the bereaved. There are a wide variety of religious traditions and you may have to acknowledge particular rites after a death. These are dealt with briefly in Chapter 59 on spiritual and religious issues.

There are various theories and outlines of what is 'normal grief', but in general, the grieving process has four basic stages, each with its own physical and emotional reactions.

Stage 1: shocked disbelief (may last up to 2 weeks)

The family will be in a state of shock when the patient dies. Physically, the bereaved may be in a state of disbelief, with deep sighing, lack of strength and appetite, choking sensations and breathlessness. These physical reactions may come in waves lasting from 20 minutes to an hour.

Emotionally, there may be a denial that the death has occurred, and a state of numbness in which there seems to be an invisible barrier between the world and the bereaved.

Stage 2: awareness develops and continues

Physically, there may be a loss of vitality and also physical symptoms of stress. Following the death of someone close, the bereaved person may develop physical symptoms similar to those shown by the deceased during his or her last illness.

Emotionally, there may be a variety of reactions, including the following:

- anger – against doctors or the hospital, other members of the family, God, or the deceased
- crying
- guilt
- hallucinations
- idealisation
- loneliness
- pining
- searching.

Stage 3: depression

After around 6 months, the bereaved may become apathetic and show a distinct lack of interest in their own life and the lives of those around them. Life may seem lacking in purpose. Existing personality or psychological problems may be exacerbated. The associated social isolation can greatly complicate the grieving process of the affected individual.

Stage 4: resolution

Eventually, the bereaved come to believe that they will cope – that they will begin to make new contacts and enjoy life again in a new way without experiencing feelings of disloyalty towards the deceased. This may take up to 1 to 2 years.

The bereaved may need permission to redevelop their social lives. They may have difficulty in knowing how to meet their friends and neighbours again. They may need permission just to take a holiday.

When a patient is bereaved, make a record in the notes. Such an entry in the notes may be important at the next consultation, or when the anniversary of the death arrives. Times of special difficulty include the following:

- birthdays (of the bereaved, the partner and the couple's children)
- Christmas or another special occasion
- holidays – planned, cancelled or taken without the deceased
- special family events (e.g. a wedding with one parent missing)
- the first anniversary of the death
- wedding anniversaries.

We are all human. We have all experienced loss to some degree, possibly in:

- broken relationships
- disappointed ambitions
- loss of our own loved ones.

Constant encounters with death and bereavement remind us of our own mortality. It is possible at any time for a particular situation to get through the chinks in the 'armour' of our professional defences. This is not a sign of weakness.

Further reading

- Blackman N. Supporting bereaved people with intellectual disabilities. *Eur J Palliat Care.* 2005; **12:** 247–8.
- Lomas D. The use of pastoral and spiritual support in bereavement care. *Nurs Times.* 2004; **100:** 34–5.
- Lyttle CP. Bereavement visiting in the community. *Eur J Palliat Care.* 2005; **12:** 74–7.
- Rolls L. UK bereavement services for children and young people. *Eur J Palliat Care.* 2005; **12:** 218–20.
- Walsh K, King M, Jones L *et al.* Spiritual beliefs may affect outcome of bereavement: prospective study. *BMJ.* 2002; **324:** 1551–4.
- Worden JW. *Grief Counselling and Grief Therapy.* London: Routledge; 1995.

Part 6

Ethical, moral and religious issues

Chapter 56

Drinking and artificial hydration (and the principles of withdrawing and withholding treatment)

Wilma O'Donnell

Appetite comes as you eat, but thirst vanishes as you drink.
François Rabelais (French physician, 1494–1553)

Introduction

As the patient becomes weaker and enters the terminal phase of their illness, they will drink less for a variety of reasons. This raises several issues and opens up an ethical debate which will be given some consideration.

Eating and drinking are basic functions that we perform every day, and which are essential for life. The family may be feeling very anxious about the patient's lack of fluid intake, and this must be remembered, and they should be made aware of how the decision is made as to whether or not to offer intravenous hydration.

C Consider

Ethics has been defined as 'the enquiry into certain situations and into the language employed to describe them'. Beauchamp and Childress[1] cite four main principles:

- autonomy – respecting other people's choices
- beneficence – acting in a way that promotes the well-being of others
- justice – treating others fairly
- non-maleficence – acting in a way that causes no harm to others.

All four principles can be applied to the question of artificial hydration in the terminally ill patient.

Consider the effects of intravenous hydration at the end of life:

- care at home may not be possible
- increased awareness, due to lowered urea levels, may increase awareness of pain
- increased respiratory and gastric secretions, which may increase vomiting
- increased urine output, possibly introducing the need for a catheter
- increased volume of effusions and ascites
- intravenous fluids may become a barrier between patient and relative.

The relatives will always obviously want the patient to die peacefully. They will benefit from being made aware of these considerations if it is deemed that an intravenous infusion is not in the best interests of the patient.

Another question arises. Is artificial hydration a medical treatment?

According to the British Medical Association,[2] all techniques that involve artificial nutrition and hydration are medical treatments, and withdrawal or withholding of either should be treated as such, but on an individual basis.

To withdraw a 'treatment' could be seen as 'passive euthanasia'.

A Assess

Why is an intravenous infusion being considered for this individual patient?

- Is the aim of the infusion to rehydrate a patient who cannot swallow liquids?
- Is it at the request of the patient or family?
- Is it at the request of other professional staff?
- Has the patient left any instruction in the form of an advance directive, stating that they do or do not wish to be given IV fluids? At the time of writing (September 2006), these are not legally binding in the UK.

The main reasons given for continuing hydration in the terminally ill are professional opinion, family opinion and personal views. Schwarte[3] believes that society has become so used to seeing intravenous fluids, etc., that it has become normal for terminally ill patients to receive intravenous fluids.

There is a common misconception among relatives that fluids are replacing food.

℞ Remedy

The symptom most commonly reported in conscious patients who are clinically dehydrated is a dry mouth. There is little evidence to suggest that giving intravenous fluids to dying patients relieves the distress of thirst.

The appropriate treatment for a dry mouth is simple mouth care. Use mouthwashes, pieces of ice to suck, or even small amounts of water from a syringe. This can be an opportunity to involve the family in the patient's care.

Discuss the options for giving fluids with the patient, the family and those caring for the patient.

An alternative to intravenous fluids, which may be appropriate for selected patients, is to give fluids subcutaneously.

With regard to intravenous and subcutaneous fluids, the following points should be borne in mind.

- They are indicated only if cognitive status is good and symptoms are controlled.
- Between 500 and 1500 ml should be given per 24 hours.
- Normal saline is the preferred fluid.
- Hyaluronidase aids the subcutaneous absorption of fluids.
- Glyceryl trinitrate (GTN) patches applied near the injection site may also assist with absorption, but may cause vasodilatory headache. They are not licensed for this use, but anecdotal reports indicate their effectiveness.
- Mobile patients can receive the treatment at night, thereby preserving daytime independence.

Decisions must be made as to whether one should use intravenous fluids to correct biochemical abnormalities such as low serum potassium levels or hypercalcaemia. Such decisions are made on an individual basis and depend on the prognosis and whether this action will benefit the patient.

The patient should be reviewed frequently and a decision made about continuing artificial hydration.

Some patients and relatives will feel that, without intravenous fluids, the patient has been left to die. The appropriate management in this situation is to discuss, openly and honestly, with the patient and their relatives any likely benefit from intravenous fluids.

Attention should be given to the need for adequate oral hygiene and mouth care.

E Extra information

The symptoms of dehydration can be distressing. Mion and O'Connell[4] and Wasylenko[5] agree that the most stressful symptoms of dehydration include confusion, headaches and dry mouth. Therefore it follows that to commence artificial hydration to relieve these symptoms would be beneficial to the patient.

Schwarte states that the main belief among both medical staff and family members is that the patient will not have any symptoms of thirst or dehydration.

Conversely, Dunlop and Ellershaw[6] feel that the benefits of not having artificial hydration far outweigh the benefits of receiving this treatment. They argue that intravenous fluids in the terminally ill patient can cause pulmonary oedema, ascites and peripheral oedema.

However, there is evidence to support the idea that patients who die without hydration die more peacefully than patients who are hydrated.

Broeckaert and Nunez-Olarte[7] concur that hydration in a sedated terminally ill patient would be considered futile within the realms of the palliative care philosophy.

Dunlop and Ellershaw state that no studies have been completed which demonstrate the adverse effects of artificial hydration, but there are many views on the futility of providing this treatment.

The 'doctrine of double effect' can also be applied here. Commencing artificial hydration in a terminally ill patient can cause discomfort, as mentioned previously, and may subsequently lead to the patient's death due to increased pulmonary oedema or infection. The intention was to hydrate the patient, not to cause discomfort or death.

The religious beliefs of patients, families and staff play a huge part in how they morally justify the decisions that are made. Brett and Jersild[8] state that Christian patients and families often demand aggressive treatment and fluids at the end of life, as they are either hoping for miracles or don't want to give up on God. However, Vere[9], writing on behalf of the Christian Medical Fellowship, lists 10 key points for guiding medical staff with regard to withdrawal of fluids and treatment. One of these points is that 'Doctors tend to over-treat towards the end of life, causing demand for euthanasia'.

The Roman Catholic Church's argument is that death is God's way. They do not agree with euthanasia but do agree that death cannot be prevented. Craig[10] believes that when death is imminent, suggestions can be made to Catholic families that it is time to hand their loved one over to God. This type of conversation may prevent any thoughts of continuing, or commencing, artificial hydration when the benefits to the patient would be minimal.

In 2004, the General Medical Council stated that 'life has a natural end' and that this should be allowed.

However, in a study by Rietjens *et al.*[11] in the Netherlands, it was felt that patients had a more comfortable death without hydration.

Relatives of Jewish patients, who believe that life should be preserved for as long as possible, regardless of its quality, may request that intravenous fluids are given, even to comatose patients.[12]

Islam regards life as sacred, and anything that is seen to hasten death will be resisted. It is important for Muslim patients and relatives to be made fully aware of the effects of offering or withdrawing intravenous fluids in the terminal stage of illness.[13]

With regard to withdrawing and withholding treatment, the European Court of Human Rights has ruled that it could be 'burdensome' if doctors had to apply to the High Court every time they wished to end a life by withdrawing food and water.[14]

References

1 Beachmamp TL, Childress JF. *Principles of Biomedical Ethics.* 5th ed. Oxford: Oxford University Press; 2001. p. 12.

2 British Medical Association. *Withholding and Withdrawing Life-prolonging Medical Treatment: guidance for decision making.* London: BMJ Books; 1999.

3 Schwarte A. Ethical decisions regarding nutrition and the terminally ill. *Gastroenterol Nurs.* 2001; **24:** 29–33.

4 Mion LC, O'Connell A. Parenteral hydration and nutrition in the geriatric patient: clinical and ethical issues. *J Infus Nurs.* 2003; **26:** 144–52.

5 Wasylenko E. *Hydration and Palliative Care. Clinical pearls from continuing care medicine rounds.* 2001. Available on Calgary Health Region website: www.calgaryhealthregion.ca/clin/cme/ccmed/pearls/ltcp0101.pdf

6 Dunlop RJ, Ellershaw JE. On withholding nutrition and hydration in the terminally ill: has palliative medicine gone too far? *J Med Ethics.* 1995; **21:** 141.

7 Broeckaert B, Nunez-Olarte JM. Sedation in palliative care: facts and concepts. In: Ten Hav H, Clark D, editors. *The Ethics of Palliative Care: European perspectives.* Buckingham: Open University Press; 2002.

8 Brett Allan S, Jersild P. 'Inappropriate' treatment near the end of life: conflict between religious convictions and clinical judgement. *Arch Intern Med.* 2003; **163:** 1645–9.

9 Vere D. *When to Withdraw or Withhold Treatment.* Christian Medical Fellowship Files Number 7. London: Christian Medical Fellowship; 1999.

10 Craig G. Terminal sedation. *Catholic Medical Quarterly* February, 2002.

11 Rietjens JAC, van der Heide A, Vrakking AM *et al.* Physician reports of terminal sedation without hydration or nutrition for patients nearing death in the Netherlands. *Ann Intern Med.* 2004; **141:** 178–85.

12 Spitzer J. *Caring for Jewish Patients.* Oxford: Radcliffe Medical Press; 2003. p. 147.

13 Sheikh A, Gatrad AR. *Caring for Muslim Patients.* Oxford: Radcliffe Medical Press; 2000.

14 *Image News*, September 2006, p. 2. Manchester: Coverdale Centre; www.imagenet.org.uk

Further reading

- Antoun S. Artificial nutrition at the end of life: is it justified? *Eur J Palliat Care.* 2006; **13:** 194–7.
- Claisse L, Grosshans C, Passadori Y. The use of hypodermoclysis in palliative care. *Eur J Palliat Care.* 2005; **12:** 243–6.
- Das A. The value of an ethics history? *J R Soc Med.* 2005; **98:** 262–6.
- Dimond B. Legal issues concerning the withholding of feeding from patients. *Nurs Times.* 2004; **100:** 56–9.
- General Medical Council. Withholding life-prolonging treatments: debating the ethics (feature article). *Your GMC.* 2006; **7:** 8–9.
- Markwell H. End of life: a Catholic view. *Lancet.* 2005; **366:** 1132–5.
- Panting G. Making decisions on withholding or withdrawing treatment. *Guidelines Pract.* 2005; **8:** 43–4.
- Paternoster B, Burucoa B. Ethical questions at the end of life. *Eur J Palliat Care.* 2003; **10:** 16–19.
- Radbruch L, Pestinger M. Müller A *et al.* Antibiotics and palliative care. *Eur J Palliat Care.* 2006; **13:** 5–9.
- Sensky T. Withdrawal of life-sustaining treatment. *BMJ.* 2002; **325:** 175–6.

Chapter 57

Refusing more treatment

> Every hospital should have a plaque in the physicians' and students' entrances: 'There are some patients we cannot help; there are none we cannot harm.'
>
> Arthur L Bloomfield (1888–1962), in a personal communication written following an iatrogenic tragedy

Introduction

The decision not to accept any more treatment often arises from misunderstandings or erroneous ideas and beliefs with regard to the safety of the drugs used. This may include fears of addiction to morphine, or the relatives' mistaken belief that effective symptom control will cause loss of consciousness, resulting in loss of contact with the patient and possible premature death.[1]

It may be best if the reasons for the decision to refuse further treatment are explored by a suitably qualified member of staff who is not involved in treating the patient. Introducing a new person often allows the patient to feel that they can ask the questions they need answered, but some patients may question why a new team member is involved, and this should be carefully explained. A member of staff who is not personally involved may be better equipped to explore the patient's fears and deal with them.

If, after being thoroughly appraised of the options and the effects and side-effects of the treatments available, a patient decides to discontinue treatment, the family should be offered extra support to help them to come to terms with this decision.

C Consider

Why does the patient wish to have no more treatment? Has there been any previous indication that they might not wish to accept any particular treatment? If so, how was this situation addressed?

The patient might be depressed and have lost the will to live. They might have experienced seeing a loved one die in pain or with his or her symptoms poorly controlled in the era when palliative care was not a well-developed specialty. Such memories are long-lived, and patients may not appreciate what is possible now with new drugs and modern palliative care services.

A Assess

By careful and sensitive discussion, find out whether the patient or the relatives have misunderstandings and fears about the disease and the treatment options available.

- Has the patient lost hope?
- Is the patient becoming depressed and losing the will to live?

- Do they fear a lingering painful death and think that refusing treatment might speed things up or give them more 'control'? They might not appreciate that most symptoms can be controlled and a reasonable quality of life maintained.

Gently explore whether they have memories of a 'bad death'.

What are the thoughts and fears of the patient's family?

℞ Remedy

Take a careful history from the patient, exploring the reasons for their decision and making it clear that they are not under any obligation to accept any treatment.

Assure the patient that the hoped for benefits and likely side-effects of any treatment offered will be honestly explained to them, and that the final decision about what they accept rests with them.

Review all of the treatments that are currently being prescribed, explaining why these are being offered and what they are intended to do. Find out about any side-effects or symptoms that the patient may have experienced, and assess whether these are actually due to the treatment or part of the disease process. If an alternative medication is available, invite the patient to try this, encouraging them to feel that they have a choice and are allowed to report any problems which they experience with any drug offered.

Ask about the patient's past experience of any treatment that they do not wish to continue. Have they obtained information from other sources? They may have been searching the Internet or been given information from a source that was unreliable or that they misunderstood.

Are other treatment options available? If so, explain what these are.

Allow the patient adequate time to consider all of the options and arrange a further discussion, at an agreed time, but offering to be available to answer any questions.

Offer to be available for further discussion with the patient's relatives, with their consent and with the patient present if he or she so wishes.

Whatever course of action is chosen, review the decision regularly and check that the patient has not changed his or her mind.

E Extra information

The fears concerning treatment, especially high doses of opioids, are often unfounded, and result from poor communication or misunderstandings. A paper published in the journal *Cancer*[2], reports that high doses of morphine do not hasten death in the terminally ill. Patt and Lang[3] state that 'misconceptions about the effects and side-effects of morphine are the primary reason why people with cancer around the world are undermedicated'.

Some of the unfounded fears that patients express about the use of strong opioids are as follows.

- The use of morphine means that the doctors are running out of options for treating pain.
- One will become addicted to the morphine.
- Morphine, if used 'too early', will not work as effectively later on.

- Pain means that disease is progressing, and therefore one is better to suffer in silence.
- Taking morphine will result in one losing control.

In addition, some patients try to 'monitor' their disease progression by assessing their pain and how well it is responding to the doses of analgesia that are being given. They often fail to appreciate how many factors influence pain perception, and attribute their pain severity to disease status alone.

Some doctors still have a poor knowledge of the use of opioids in the terminally ill.[4] Patients may have bad memories of poor care given to older family members when they were terminally ill, and think that this is what will happen to them. This is usually the result of poor communication, and can usually be addressed by giving a full explanation of the drugs and modern treatments used. Anticipate the common responses, anxieties and misunderstandings, and dispel unrealistic fears about drug tolerance, addiction and uncontrolled side-effects.

Let the patient know that you will be available to listen to what they want to say, and that you are always available to honestly discuss any fears they have about their treatment.

Probably the most commonly encountered treatment refusal is that of blood transfusions by Jehovah's Witnesses. Most Jehovah's Witnesses will either be carrying a card or will happily sign the standard form used by most hospitals. This releases you from responsibility for the outcome of such a refusal. The card carried by some Witnesses directs that no blood should be given, and is signed by the patient and two witnesses, one of whom is usually a family member and the second a congregation elder or a solicitor, both of whom are authorised to uphold this decision in the event that the patient cannot express his or her own wishes.

As new artificial blood products become available, the Watchtower Society, which is the authoritative body governing the Jehovah's Witnesses movement, has issued new guidance, and this has been updated and may change as new instructions are issued by the Watchtower Society.

You are advised to ask the patient or an elder from the local Kingdom Hall for current advice if the situation is unclear.

References

1 Azoulay D Brajtman S, Yehezkel M *et al.* When the family demands the discontinuation of morphine. *Eur J Palliat Care.* 2000; 7: 138–40.

2 Bercovitch M, Adunsky A. Patterns of high-dose morphine use in a home-care hospice service: Should we be afraid of it? *Cancer.* 2004; **101:** 1477–7

3 Patt RB, Lang SS. *The Complete Guide to Relieving Cancer Pain and Suffering,* New York: Oxford University Press; 2004. p. 135.

4 Valera J-P, Aubry R. Morphine – doctors' beliefs and the myths. *Eur J Palliat Care.* 2000; **7:** 178–82.

Further reading

- Haas F. Understanding the legal implications of living wills. *Nurs Times.* 2005; **101:** 34–7.
- Kacen L, Madjar I, Denham J *et al.* Patients deciding to forgo or stop active treatment for cancer. *Eur J Palliat Care.* 2005; **12:** 108–11.
- Panting G. How does a living will affect the care you give your patient? *Guidelines Pract.* 2004; **7:** 58–60.

Chapter 58

Resuscitation

> I am also satisfied that a person who has a duty to care may be guilty of murder by omitting to fulfil that duty, as much as by committing any positive act.
>
> Lord Havers (British lawyer and politician, 1923–1992), in a High Court judgement in 1982

Introduction

Stedman's Medical Dictionary defines cardiac arrest as 'complete cessation of cardiac activity – either electric, mechanical, or both'.[1]

I remember vividly the first resuscitation attempt I saw as a student nurse: I was shocked by the noise, the drama, the urgency and the brutality.[2]

In April 2000, Age Concern stated that decisions not to resuscitate were made to alleviate the bed crisis within the NHS. All that is achieved by statements like this is that people become unnerved and confused by the issues surrounding 'do not attempt resuscitation' (DNAR) orders and euthanasia. Statements like this have made it difficult for staff to make the decision as to whether to resuscitate or not.

The outcome of cardiopulmonary resuscitation (CPR) can be poor at times. It is affected by disease, but not necessarily by age.

The public perception of CPR, possibly based on televised hospital programmes designed for entertainment, is probably over-optimistic about the outcome. However, modern medicine still has its limits.

The Patient's Charter published in 1991 states that the consumer is entitled to respect as an individual.[3]

On admission to hospital, patients are not always medically or mentally fit enough to be able to state their wishes with regard to care, or indeed when treatment should stop. This is when advance directives and living wills are beneficial. When a person is considering using these, they should be prepared, with medical supervision, to ensure that the patient knows exactly what he is consenting to or opting out of. Discussions with a relative about what you would or would not want in hospital are not ideal. Legally, relatives have no right to decide whether a patient should be resuscitated or not. Therefore, although they can say what they *think* the patient would like, and hopefully this would be taken into consideration by the consultant, the ultimate decision would lie with the consultant.

CPR is the only medical intervention that presumes patient consent. If there is no realistic chance of survival, then not attempting CPR should not be seen as depriving the patient of life.

C Consider

In 2001, the Resuscitation Council (UK) published expert advice on the subject of advance DNAR orders.[4]

After conducting a clinical assessment, it may be appropriate to consider making a DNAR order in the following circumstances.

- CPR is not expected to restart the patient's heart and breathing.
- Restarting the patient's heart and breathing will confer no benefit.
- The anticipated burdens outweigh the expected benefit.

A DNAR order is specific to CPR. It does not imply that other treatment will be withdrawn, but this fear has been recorded.[5,6]

It is hard for relatives to decide whether to attempt to resuscitate or not – after all, we do not see clearly when our eyes are full of tears.

When being asked to make the decision, do they want an end to the suffering of their loved one, or do they want to keep them alive in the hope that a treatment for a terminal illness becomes available? If they choose not to have the patient resuscitated, is this a form of euthanasia or physician-assisted suicide? These are real fears, and they should not be dismissed as unfounded or unimportant. The relatives will be living with these worries long after you have moved on.

Before entering into discussion with the patient and their relatives, the staff must have a good knowledge of the prognosis, the likely outcome of CPR and the quality of life that the patient is likely to have if CPR is successful.

It must be recognised that families may be of the opinion that successful resuscitation offers the hope that, if the patient is kept alive, then perhaps cure will be possible. The fact is that, following resuscitation, the patient is often much more poorly. Families need to be gently but realistically made aware of this fact.

Negative predictors of survival include cancer, especially if it is advanced or metastatic.[7]

The following suggestions have been made.

- Literature should be available for patients, their families and carers, offering information about CPR, how decisions are made and how they may be involved in this decision-making process.[4]
- Decisions relating to CPR must be communicated clearly to all staff.[4]
- The unit CPR policy should be published and easily accessible by anyone who wishes to consult it, including patients, family members or other carers.[8]

A Assess

The word 'euthanasia' comes from two Greek words (*eu* and *thanatos*), which translate in English as 'good death'. The real meaning of the word is lost, and now means assisting to die. The following questions have to be considered. Are we attempting resuscitation of the patient for them to continue suffering? Can their pain be adequately controlled? Can we provide good symptom relief? Are they going to get better? Or is a cardiac arrest considered a 'good death' in the circumstances?

Edwards wrote in 1996 that 'One form of euthanasia is passive euthanasia, which involves bringing about a person's death by omission'.[9] There is no doubt that DNAR orders are an act of omission which leads to patient death.

Euthanasia is not legal in the UK. Therefore it has to be made very clear why the decision not to attempt resuscitation has been made, and this must be clearly documented.

The United Kingdom Central Council for Nursing, Midwifery and Health Visiting (UKCC) code of professional conduct states that no act or omission on our part should be detrimental to patients. It also requires nurses to be accountable for their own practice, and to ensure that their skills and knowledge are maintained and that they are practising safely.[10]

The UKCC also states that nurses will accept the role of advocate for the patient.[11]

Advocacy is concerned with the well-being and interests of patients.[10]

The whole subject of DNAR orders is a moral minefield. There are various aspects that can affect the decision as to whether or not to attempt to resuscitate.

The Human Rights Act (1998) states that everyone has:

- the right to life (Article 2)
- the right to be free from inhuman or degrading treatment (Article 3)
- the right to freedom of expression, which includes the right to hold opinions and receive information (Article 10)
- the right to be free from discriminatory practices (Article 14).

These should all be taken into account when making a decision about resuscitation.

Legally, not to resuscitate a patient who has not consented to a DNAR order could be seen as a neglect of duty, but to attempt resuscitation on a patient who has not given consent to attempted resuscitation is technically assault!

'The principle of double effect is an action which has a good objective, and may be performed despite the fact that the objective can only be achieved at the expense of a coincident harmful effect.'[12] This means that to give pain relief in high doses to a terminally ill patient, which simultaneously shortens their life, may be ethically right, but to give the same high dose to a patient who has similar pain but stands a good chance of recovery would be wrong.

If the decision is made not to attempt resuscitation on a patient, could it be regarded as demonstrating the doctrine of double effect? Or should it be seen as the slippery slope, posing a threat to vulnerable members of our society, in view of the fact that DNAR orders are issued more often for elderly patients, with malignancy, dementia, pneumonia and stroke?

'When considering mortality in people aged 65 and over, the most common cause continues to be heart disease (32%), followed by cancer (23%), cerebrovascular disease (14%) and respiratory disease (12%).'[13] So could it be that the DNAR orders were issued because of the debilitation caused by the disease and not because of the patient's age, which was purely coincidental?

In 1997, Mason and McCall Smith[14] considered other ethical issues, namely:

- autonomy – the patient's wishes should be respected, and not to involve a patient in the decision about resuscitation negates their autonomy
- utility – whether an action is right or wrong is judged by its outcome
- non-maleficence – 'experience shows that acting in the patient's best interest does not necessarily mean that life should be preserved regardless of quality'.

These issues should be considered in CPR decisions in all age groups. Age alone should not be a factor.

The *British Medical Journal*[15] published the results of a questionnaire issued to 80 hospital doctors on patient resuscitation. Only one of the 34 doctors who returned the questionnaire thought that patients should be consulted about CPR,

33 doctors thought that patients should not be consulted, and 24 senior staff would not resuscitate healthy patients over the age of 70 years.

℞ Remedy

Resuscitation may not always be the best option. Life should not necessarily be prolonged at all costs.[16]

As cardiac arrest is often sudden and unexpected, should decisions be made on a patient's admission to hospital? Should patients be told all about CPR – exactly what it is and how it is carried out – and be allowed to make an informed decision?

'The patient or carer can only make an informed choice if he or she is given clear information at every stage of care.'[10]

It is considered unethical to issue a DNAR order without consultation with the patient.

If a patient is considered unsuitable for CPR, this does not exclude them from all treatments. Therefore if they have a condition that could lead to cardiac arrest, treatment should be carried out, up to the point of their heart stopping.[4]

According to a joint statement issued by the British Medical Association, the Resuscitation Council (UK) and the Royal College of Nursing, any area that may be involved in attempting resuscitation should have local policies in place to aid decision making. The guidelines issued by them are to assist in setting up local policies for advanced decisions, which form part of the patient's care plan. They go on to say that written information regarding resuscitation policies should be given to patients along with other literature provided about the healthcare establishment.

It is also stated that DNAR orders should be a multi-disciplinary decision. Any decision regarding CPR should be documented, signed and dated in the patient's notes.

Cultural and religious influences also need to be taken into account. The Catechism of the Catholic Church, under the fifth commandment, states that 'Life and physical health are precious gifts entrusted to us by God',[17] but it is acceptable to discontinue inappropriate medical treatment, and good palliative care should be encouraged.

We have already noted that Article 10 of the Human Rights Act 1998 states that people have the right to receive information. The UKCC guidelines for professional practice state that 'Communication is an essential part of good practice'.

The new joint guidelines on resuscitation state that patients should be given information on resuscitation on admission to hospital. One needs to consider whether this is the most appropriate time to be giving this information. Would it be offputting for a patient who has been admitted for a routine procedure to receive leaflets on CPR? How will patients who are admitted for end-of-life care view this information? Will it engender false hope of a longer survival?

Patients and relatives do need to be aware that in certain situations CPR is just drawing out the death process, especially if the patient is in the terminal phase of their illness.

The goals of palliative care are as follows:

- achievement of the best possible quality of life for patients and their families
- good control of symptoms

- to facilitate adjustment to the many 'losses' of advanced and terminal illness
- to facilitate and guide completion of 'unfinished business'
- a dignified death, with minimum distress, in the patient's place of choice
- prevention of problems in bereavement.

In attempts to maintain life at all costs, are we losing the ability to provide good palliative care for people with terminal diseases? Where do we stop fighting death and ease it? 'Terminally ill people are those with active and progressive disease for which curative treatment is not possible or not appropriate and from which death can reasonably be expected within 12 months' (*Care of People with Terminal Illness*, National Association of Health Authorities and Trusts, 1991; EL (95) 22, NHS Executive 23 February 1995; and *Specialist Palliative Care: A Statement of Definitions*, National Council for Hospice and Specialist Palliative Care Service, 1995).

This time needs to be clearly defined for patients and their relatives, so that they have time to prepare for death and to say their goodbyes, without the continuing false hope that the patient's life can be saved.

Staff also need to recognise that the patient is dying and that resuscitation is not always appropriate. Everyone in the team needs to be agreed about this. There is a need to develop a decision-making tool that would support staff in the diagnosis of dying.[18]

Campbell[18] concludes that the four main themes that influence end-of-life decision making by nursing and medical staff within the hospital environment are *caring, respect, communication*and *knowledge*. These decisions are made within the four domains of health – physical, psychological, social and spiritual – when staff are planning end-of-life care for their patients.

Equally, 'blanket' DNAR orders should not be tolerated, as people with conditions such as malignancies could be living relatively symptom free and may be suitable for resuscitation attempts.

E Extra information

> Any attempts at CPR must be competent and in accordance with established clinical guidelines.[4]

Now that these new guidelines are in place, we have to ensure that they are being applied correctly and that they are being applied to all patients.

Reasons why patients might not discuss resuscitation include the following:[19]

- inability to read the information
- lack of privacy (e.g. presence of visitors)
- language barriers and no translator present
- personal choice not to discuss the subject.

Clinical governance is an umbrella term used to look at improving patient care through evidence-based practice, clinical audit, risk management and professional development. It should be a multi-disciplinary approach involving clinical staff, management and patients.

References

1 *Stedman's Medical Dictionary.* 28th edition. Philadelphia, PA: Lippincott, Williams & Wilkins; 2005.
2 Chellel A. *Resuscitation.* Edinburgh: Churchill Livingston; 2000.
3 Chenitz WC, Stone JT, Salisbury SA, editors. *Gerontology.* Philadelphia, PA: WB Saunders Company; 1991.
4 Resuscitation Council (UK). *Decisions Relating to Cardiopulmonary Resuscitation: a joint statement from the British Medical Association, the Resuscitation Council (UK) and the Royal College of Nursing.* London: Resuscitation Council (UK); 2001.
5 Daly B, Gorecki J, Sadowski A *et al.* Do-not-resuscitate practices in the chronically critically ill. *Heart Lung.* 1996; **25:** 310–17.
6 Jezewski MA. Do-not-resuscitate status: conflict and culture brokering in critical care units. *Heart Lung.* 1994; 23: 391–6.
7 Newman R. Developing guidelines for resuscitation in terminal care. *Eur J Palliat Care.* 2002; **9:** 60–63.
8 Department of Health. *Resuscitation Policy.* Service Circular HSC2000/028. London: Department of Health; 2000.
9 Edwards SD. *Nursing Ethics: a principle-based approach.* Chippenham: Anthony Rowe Ltd; 1996.
10 United Kingdom Central Council for Nursing, Midwifery and Health Visiting (UKCC). *Guidelines for Professional Practice.* London: UKCC; 1996.
11 Duxbury J. Mental health. In: Walsh M, editor. *Watson's Clinical Nursing and Related Sciences.* 5th ed. London: Baillière Tindall; 2000.
12 Mason JK, McCall Smith A. *Law and Medical Ethics.* 5th ed. London: Butterworths; 1999.
13 Redfern SJ, Ross FM. *Nursing Older People.* London: Churchill Livingstone; 1999.
14 Mason JK, McCall Smith A. *Law and Medical Ethics*, 4th ed. London: Butterworths; 1994.
15 Hill ME, MacQuillan G, Forsyth M, Heath DA. Cardiopulmonary resuscitation: who makes the decision? *BMJ.* 1994; **308:** 1677.
16 British Medical Association. *Decisions Relating to Cardiopulmonary Resuscitation: a joint statement from the British Medical Association, the Resuscitation Council (UK) and the Royal College of Nursing.* London: British Medical Association; 2001.
17 *Catechism of the Catholic Church.* Dublin: Veritas; 1994.
18 Campbell S. *Exploring Nursing and Medical Decision Making at the End of Life in Palliative Care within the Hospital Setting.* MSc dissertation, Queen Margaret University College, Edinburgh, 2006.
19 Fidler H, Thompson C, Freeman A *et al.* Barriers to implementing a policy not to attempt resuscitation in acute medical admissions: prospective cross-sectional study of a successive cohort. *BMJ.* 2006; **332:** 461–2.

Further reading

- Ackroyd R. Medically futile resuscitation: can it ever be justified? *Eur J Palliat Care.* 2005; **12:** 207–9.
- Conroy SP, Luxton T, Dingwall R *et al.* Cardiopulmonary resuscitation in continuing care settings: time for a rethink? *BMJ.* 2006; **332:** 479–82.
- Das A. The value of an ethics history? *J R Soc Med.* 2005; **98:** 262–6.
- Slowther A-M. Medical futility and 'Do Not Attempt Resuscitation' orders. *Clin Ethics.* 2006; **1**:18–20.

Chapter 59

Spiritual and religious issues

> We can believe what we choose. We are answerable for what we choose to believe.
>
> John H Newman (English Cardinal and theologian, 1801–1890)

Introduction

It is increasingly recognised by the nursing and medical professions that the concept of 'spirituality' is not necessarily the same as being 'religious', and goes beyond religious affiliation, seeking a meaning and purpose in life, even among those who do not believe in God.

Galanter (2006) states that 'There is no agreed definition of "spirituality." It is a way of life'.[1]

A useful working definition of spirituality is that of Murray and Zentnor:

> A quality that goes beyond religious affiliation; that strives for inspirations, reverence, awe, meaning and purpose. ... The spiritual dimension tries to be in harmony with the universe and strives for answers about the infinite, and comes into focus when the person faces emotional stress, physical illness or death.[2]

Your own definition of spirituality may not include an allegiance to any formal religion, but does the patient use the term 'spirituality' when you would refer to 'religion'? You might need to distinguish between the patient's spiritual, religious and emotional needs.

In this chapter, we shall think about both the meaning of the illness and the place of religious belief in the patient's life. Because the various religions have different beliefs and customs relating to terminal illness and death, a brief summary of the commoner religions is provided at the end of the chapter.

It is important to be aware that in these days of limited resources, some NHS trusts are considering cutting the chaplaincy input in order to save money. Palliative care nurses have commented that this will impair end-of-life care and that it also goes against the advice given in the Liverpool Care Pathway.[3]

It could also result in your being asked to advise or help, and this makes it even more important for you to have a basic knowledge of the ways in which people from different faiths approach death.

C Consider

Whether they are religious or not, many patients will be asking 'Why?' and 'Why me?'. They may be searching for a reason and a meaning for their suffering. Finding a reason may be impossible, but if they can use the illness positively, that might give it a 'meaning' and can help them to cope.

In his poem 'The Dry Salvages', T S Eliot includes the line, 'We had the experience but missed the meaning'.[4] *Perhaps that sums up your patient's feelings.*

A Assess

Is the patient seeking spiritual, emotional or religious support? What exactly is it that they are asking for? Is it help with searching for a meaning to life and the illness? Is the patient afraid to die without making peace with God?

Some patients dread a hopeless end. Others face death with endless hope and are at peace as death approaches. It is important to find out where the individual is on this 'spectrum', and what help, advice or support they need just now.

The authors recognise that you may have no religious affiliation or you may belong to a different faith from that of the patient in our multi-cultural society. Do you feel able to help? If not, who can offer appropriate advice?

It should be reasonably easy to find a minister or adviser from the patient's particular faith and ask them to visit. The patient might know whom you should contact. If not, ask the hospital or hospice chaplain, or if there is nobody to ask, the local library, Citizens Advice Bureau or the Yellow Pages might be useful resources.

℞ Remedy

Patients who are seeking spiritual guidance and comfort need to have this issue addressed as quickly as any distressing physical symptom. Many patients fear dying without making peace with (their) God, and this is an important area to address quickly when the time remaining in which to make the appropriate response is limited. It has been noted in various studies over several years that patients with a strong religious belief maintain their sense of control, hope and the meaning and purpose of life.[5]

The situation in hospitals is changing, and there is an increasing tendency for the patient to have to 'make the first move' with regard to a visit from a chaplain. Due to the recent developments and possible cuts in chaplaincy services noted above, patients may find it less easy to know how to address this issue.

Some patients wish to have a non-religious contact. They should ask the staff what arrangements they have for such a visit. Some hospitals have Spiritual Care Coordinators who visit and assess who is the best person to help with the broader issues of 'spirituality.'

In our experience, the relief and peace of mind experienced by patients who have spoken to someone about spiritual and religious issues have been obvious to family and staff alike. We therefore suggest that this is something that you should encourage and assist the patient in attending to without undue delay.

A World Health Organization Expert Committee on Palliative Care stated that patients have the right to expect that their spiritual experiences will be respected and listened to with attention.

It is possible that the patient belongs to a different religious faith from your own, and you may not be familiar with certain customs and practices that are important to them. On the following pages we have outlined some of the beliefs of the major religions. Space does not allow a detailed discussion, but a short list of other resources is included at the end.

Because the most commonly followed faith in the UK is Christianity, we have placed it first. The other religions are listed alphabetically. Where possible, quotations are included from the religious books relevant to particular religions, but in some cases it has been difficult to provide easily accessible references.

E Extra information

This is given under each religion.

Don't forget that all of the staff, you included, are also going through a stressful time caring for patients who will die, and all of you might also find it helpful to meet with a spiritual adviser at this time.

References

These references apply to the foregoing text. Additional references are listed under each religion for clarity and ease of access.

1 Galanter M. *Spirituality and the Healthy Mind: science therapy and the need for personal meaning.* Oxford: Oxford University Press; 2006.
2 Murray RB, Zentnor JB. *Nursing Concepts for Health Promotion.* London: Prentice Hall; 1989. p. 259.
3 Vere-Jones E. NHS chaplains face redundancy. *Nurs Times.* 2006; **102:** 4.
4 Eliot TS. The Dry Salvages. In: *TS Eliot Collected Poems 1909–1962.* London: Faber & Faber; 1963.
5 Koenig HG, Larson DB, Larson SS. Religion and coping with serious medical illness. *Ann Pharmacother.* 2001; **35:** 352–9.

Summary of the commoner religions

Christianity

Origin

Christianity began about 2000 years ago, and the name refers to those who follow Jesus Christ. Christianity is unique in that the Bible teaches that Jesus was crucified and died but was resurrected to life again three days later and remains alive today in Heaven. Christianity is unique in that it is the only faith that worships a living Lord Jesus Christ. The founders of all the other religions and faiths are deceased.

Books and writings

The Holy Bible (Old and New Testaments) is the basis for all the teachings of the Christian faith. The quotations used here are from the New International Version of the Bible.

Note: There are many denominations within the Christian faith, and the patient will usually prefer to see a minister from their own denomination. Most hospital chaplains will be able to offer spiritual help until the patient's preferred minister is available.

Summary of teachings

God is triune – Father, Son and Holy Spirit. Jesus Christ is the one and only Son of God and is alive today.

The *Bible* teaches that God created man (Genesis 1:27 – 'So God created man in his own image, in the image of God he created him; male and female he created them'). Christians therefore regard human life with dignity and, since it is God-given, are opposed to euthanasia, physician-assisted suicide or any act that shortens life.

The first created man, Adam, and his wife, Eve, were placed in the Garden of Eden, where Adam disobeyed God by eating forbidden fruit. As a result of Adam's disobedience (sin), everyone inherited the sinful nature. Romans 3:22–25 states that 'There is no difference, for all have sinned and fall short of the glory of God and are justified freely by his grace through the redemption that came by Christ Jesus. God presented him as a sacrifice of atonement, through faith in his blood'.

God gave the law (the Ten Commandments), but it was obvious that no one could keep the law to God's satisfaction, and a system of animal sacrifices offered on behalf of the errant sinner initially provided forgiveness. Later God sent His Son, Jesus, to die as the final sacrifice for our sins, thus offering forgiveness to anyone who believes that Jesus died for our sins, and offering us forgiveness through faith in His death for us.

The Gospel of John 3:16–18 states:

> For God so loved the world that He gave His one and only Son, that whoever believes in Him shall not perish but have eternal life. For God did not send His Son into the world to condemn the world, but to save the world through Him. Whoever believes in Him is not condemned, but whoever does not believe stands condemned already because he has not believed in the name of God's one and only Son.

Those who genuinely seek God's forgiveness through Jesus' death for their sins will receive it and go to Heaven, but those who do not ask God's forgiveness are destined to receive eternal punishment.

The Christian faith is unique in that it teaches that Jesus Christ, the one and only Son of God, died to take the punishment due to us for our sins, and was then resurrected from death. Faith in His sacrificial death guarantees forgiveness and a place in Heaven. Those who do not believe remain unforgiven and will be eternally punished in Hell.

Beliefs and traditions with regard to illness

Suffering and illness are generally accepted as the result of Adam's original sin, which affects mankind universally. Many Christians therefore do not believe that God is punishing them personally, and might see the illness as an opportunity to see God at work in their lives. They might refer to the story of Job in the Old Testament, pointing out that God allowed him to be put through extreme suffering and personal loss as an example to others of his faith in God. However, some Christians do regard illness and suffering as a personal punishment from God, and may spend time examining what they might have done wrong.

Virtually all medications are accepted and, subject to individual preference, there is usually no objection to the use of opioids. Acceptability of alcohol is an individual matter, with some strongly opposed and others prepared to accept it in moderation.

The patient might ask for representatives of their Church to read from the *Bible*, pray with them and possibly anoint them with oil as part of the Church's ministry of healing.

Terminal illness and death

There are no special preparations for death or after death. Burial and cremation are acceptable (some denominations are less accepting of cremation), and there is generally no objection to a post-mortem examination of the body.

Baha'i

Origin

The Baha'i faith originated in Iran in the nineteenth century and is based on the teachings of Mizra Hussayn Ali Nuri, known to his followers as Baha'u'llah (Glory of God). He declared himself to be the manifestation of God who was to lead mankind to peace and unity, and to overcome the differences between the various religions that traditionally disagreed in their teaching. Baha'u'llah taught that God's plan is for a single language, currency and administrative body that will bring about universal peace and harmony.

Books and writings

The Baha'i patient may request a copy of the Baha'i prayer book and other Baha'i literature. If the patient cannot supply details of a Baha'i representative, the group may be contacted by referring to the telephone directory. (If no local group is listed, the London headquarters can give advice. Tel: 020 7584 2566. Email: nsa@bahai.org.uk).

Summary of teachings

Baha'is teach that God is one person, not three as taught by the *Bible*.

Baha'is believe that Jesus Christ is not the unique Son of God, but one of many prophets. They believe that Jesus' death is not particularly significant and is not a sacrifice for our sin. Baha'is believe that the *Bible* is incomplete without the writings of the Baha'u'llah, and that the teachings of Christianity have now been surpassed by their new revelations.

Baha'is believe that there is a Divine remedial judgement after death, but no eternal punishment for unbelievers.

Beliefs and traditions with regard to illness and treatment

Drugs are allowed, if prescribed. Alcohol and narcotics (drugs like morphine) are forbidden, but if two doctors confirm that there is no alternative available, or that the alcohol is an essential ingredient of a medication, they can be given.

Terminal illness and death

Patients will either recite Baha'i prayers or have them read if they are unable to recite for themselves.

After death, the body is washed and wrapped in silk or cotton. A special ring is placed on the finger, and the body is placed in a coffin made of fine hard wood, stone or crystal.

Cremation is forbidden, and burial should take place within one hour's journey of the place of death.

Buddhism

Note: There are several schools within Buddhism, and this information is very general.

Origin

There is some uncertainty about the Buddha, but it is generally accepted that Siddhartha Gautama, the Buddha or 'Awakened One', was born in 566 BC and died in 486 BC.

Siddhartha Gautama is traditionally reported to have been of royal birth. One day, when he visited a park outside the palace, he saw three things that made him confront the reality of death, namely a sick man, an old man and a corpse. On returning to the palace he met a man who had renounced ordinary life in favour of extreme abstinence and self-denial, and these 'Four Sights' inspired Siddhartha Gautama to follow a life of renunciation.

Initially the Buddha lived an ascetic existence, but after a period of time he decided that such extreme self-discipline was not satisfactory and, after a prolonged period of intense meditation, he gained insight into the Four Noble Truths, which are the core of Buddhist teachings.

Books and writings

The Buddha's teachings on truth, order, righteousness, duty and justice (dharma) were not written down during his lifetime, and it was around 350 years later that Buddhist monks met to try to preserve his teachings. After initial agreement, divisions and differences emerged that have resulted in the different schools of Buddhism.

One useful website is www.chezpaul.org.uk/buddhism/uk/index.htm.

Summary of teachings

Buddhism teaches the 'Four Noble Truths', which can be summarised as follows.

1 All living things are characterised by suffering and unhappiness.
2 It is wrong desire and selfishness that cause this suffering.
3 If one removes wrong desire and selfishness then one eliminates suffering and unhappiness.
4 The way to remove wrong desire and selfishness is to adhere to the eightfold path to enlightenment.

Buddhist teaching is based on non-violence, brotherhood and hard work. Buddhists believe in reincarnation, so that after death one goes on to another life, progressing towards infinite perfection or *nirvana*. *Karma*, the balance of merit and demerit accumulated by an individual during their lifetime, determines the nature of their next reincarnation.

Buddhists believe that someone who accumulates good *karma* in life will be reborn into a more favourable position in a future life. The opposite also applies, so that those who perform bad actions will have to eradicate those negative merits by spending a period of time in Hell, the severity of punishment that they receive being ranked according to the seriousness of their demerits.

Those in Hell can wipe out their sins and be reborn into humanity, but conversely, even when one has reached the highest state of reincarnation, one can slip and be reincarnated at a lower level. Even those who rise to become a god can exhaust their merit and return as a mere human. No state of reincarnation is permanent.

Nirvana is a state in which one ceases to achieve *karma*, is free of all desire and ignorance, and achieves liberation from the endless cycle of death and rebirth. To achieve *nirvana*, total selflessness is essential, with an absence of separateness and suffering. One must follow the Noble Eightfold Path, which arises from the Four Noble Truths that lead man to enlightenment through his effort.

The Noble Eightfold Path consists of 'right understanding', 'right thought', 'right speech', 'right action', 'right livelihood', 'right effort', 'right mindfulness' and 'right concentration'.

After death, Buddhists expect to be reincarnated until they eventually reach *nirvana*.

> When I attain this highest perfect wisdom, I will deliver all sentient beings into the eternal peace of nirvana.
>
> The Buddha, quoted in the *Diamond Sutta*

Beliefs and traditions with regard to illness

Suffering is the outcome of desire. If desire had truly been extinguished and the patient had truly wanted nothing, there would have been no suffering.

The patient might wish to have a small statue of the Buddha with them. They will want time for uninterrupted meditation several times during the day. The times are not fixed and the duration of meditation is a matter of personal choice.

The lotus flower (a water lily with its roots in mud) is a common image in Buddhist teachings. It symbolises the belief that enlightenment (the flower) can be achieved during human suffering (the mud).

Buddhists will consent to all treatment in the palliative care context. Buddhism stresses the relief of suffering and pain in particular, but the patient may be concerned that morphine and similar drugs might cloud their mind. Buddhism strongly emphasises the importance of 'mindfulness' and awareness of everything. The patient should be reassured that spiritual awareness should still be possible when morphine and other strong painkillers are correctly prescribed, but if they refuse these drugs after a full explanation has been offered, their wishes must be respected. Some medications will cause unavoidable drowsiness, and the wishes of the patient must be considered if these drugs are considered necessary to control symptoms such as anxiety or agitation.

Terminal illness and death

As mentioned previously, there are different schools of Buddhism. If possible, a Buddhist monk from the same school of Buddhism should visit. The Buddhist Society in London can supply contact details. (Tel: 0845 458 4716; lines open 10am–5pm Monday to Friday.)

Pure Land Buddhism holds that if a believer chants, in full faith, the name of the celestial Buddha, then the Buddha will visit at the point of death and transport the dying person to the 'Pure Land', where they can prepare for *nirvana,* freed from all earthly distractions.

In Japanese Zen Buddhism there is a tradition of composing a poem at the moment of death.

Buddhist funerals are designed to assist the deceased to a better birth. Buddhist texts may be read in the presence of the corpse and afterwards in front of a picture of the deceased. Various Buddhas are portrayed in the texts, and the deceased person is believed to be able to unite with these over a period of up to 49 days, which is considered to be the time required for the person to be transformed to their new life.

Cremation is traditional.

Further reading on Buddhism

- Eckel MD. *Understanding Buddhism.* London: Duncan Baird Publishers; 2003.

Chinese religions (Buddhism, Confucianism, Taoism and folk religion)

Chinese religion is not a single belief system, but is made up of four main elements – Buddhism, Confucianism, Taoism and folk religion. The rituals of one of these may be mixed freely with the ceremonies of another.

Buddhism

Buddhism came to China in the first century AD and influenced the development of Confucianism and Taoism.

Confucius, Lao-tzu and the Buddha all lived at around the same time, and these religions may have coexisted in China.

A more detailed discussion of Buddhism is given above.

Confucianism

Confucianism takes its name from Confucius, who lived from 551 to 479 BC. He encouraged worship of one's ancestors and taught that people should respect their parents and show kindness to humanity. Confucius was not a prophet, but a travelling teacher who taught that people should practise kindness and respect. Several writings show that he concentrated on the responsibilities of this life rather than speculating on the hereafter.

Divination is an important part of Confucianism, and texts like the *I Ching* (*Book of Changes*) are among the classic texts.

Confucianism is primarily concerned with one's moral conduct on earth, but does include a spiritual dimension in that Confucius taught that mankind is guided by a higher authority which he called 'Heaven.' Early on it was taught that Heaven approved of harmony, which came to be seen as a balance between two forces – *yin* and *yang.*

Confucianism teaches that everything is composed of *Qi,* the vital matter from which everything is made.

Yin is that part of *Qi* which is dark, feminine and quiescent. *Yang,* on the other hand, is light, masculine and mobile.

Those who have died now reside in a spirit world and consist of *Qi*. Everyone is believed to have at least two souls, namely a *hun* soul made of *yang* and a *po* soul made of *yin*. At death, the *hun* soul ascends, as it is made of *yang,* and the *po* soul, which is made of *yin*, descends into the ground and remains with the body as long as it is properly buried and maintained by grave rites and offerings.

The *po* soul is also believed to descend to hell, where it is judged for its sins and eventually reincarnated. Through good works and offerings, the family can speed the passage of loved ones through Hell.

Unhappy ancestors are believed to be the cause of ill-health and misfortune.

Euthanasia and physician-assisted suicide

A modern-day Confucian could agree that a person can end his or her life, and a doctor can ethically participate in that ending, if and only if that decision is the product of careful and searching deliberation among all relevant close relatives. A person could not take such a decision in isolation. If some family members had strong reservations, then perhaps there should be a waiting period in deference to that objection.

Further reading on Confucianism

- Oldstone-Moore J. *Understanding Confucianism*. London: Duncan Baird Publishers; 2003.

Taoism

Taoism was founded by Lao-tzu in the sixth century BC. *Tao* means 'the way', and it is reached through meditation, chanting and physical exercise, which are believed to achieve immortality. Little is known about Lao-tzu, but the main Taoist text, *Tao-te-Ching* (*Classic of the Way and its Power*) is attributed to him.

Taoism teaches that the earth's natural forces (*ch'i*) are made up two components, *yin* and *yang*. Through a correct balance of *yin* and *yang* one can achieve a healthy state of mind. By following the Tao, one can obtain long life and immortality. Immortality is interpreted in two ways – first, eternal life in a new body, and secondly and more symbolically, a release from the worries of everyday life.

To achieve harmony of *yin* and *yang*, a complex mixture of rituals has evolved. This includes meditation, chanting, physical exercise and natural medicines. Illness is believed to be due to an imbalance of *yin* and *yang*, and the balance can be restored by use of acupuncture, which is believed to control the flow of vital energy in invisible channels in the body.

There are two types of soul, namely a *hun* soul made of *yang ch'i* and a *p'o* soul made of *yin ch'i*. At death, the *hun* soul ascends, as it is made of *yang*, and the *p'o* soul, which is made of *yin*, descends into the ground. Funeral rituals are performed to settle the *p'o* soul into ancestral tablets kept on the domestic altar in the home, and to ensure the peaceful settling of the *p'o* soul into the grave.

Taoist priests are important, and are hired by the family to prepare the documents necessary to be offered to the bureaucrats of the underworld to ensure that the deceased person spends a minimal time suffering for any misdeeds committed during his or her life. A writ of pardon may be sent at the funeral ceremony.

The Taoist priest also has an important role in communicating with the dead person and restoring harmony within the family. After burial, the family must bring things needed by the dead person, namely food, drink, spirit money and any other necessity.

Euthanasia and physician-assisted suicide

A philosophic Taoist of the Chuang Tzu variety, at least, would probably be opposed to euthanasia and physician-asssisted suicide. Why intervene? If death is coming, as it is, ultimately, for all of us, why hurry the process along or slow it down? Palliative care would be acceptable from a Taoist viewpoint, but not active suicide.

Further reading on Taoism

- Oldstone-Moore J. *Understanding Taoism.* London: Duncan Baird Publishers; 2003.

Folk religions

Folk religions involve the worship of a variety of gods originating in various myths and legends.

In ancient times, farmers believed that heavenly spirits controlled the sun and rain. It became popular to believe that the spirits of deceased ancestors could possibly intervene to ensure better crops.

A number of domestic gods thus developed over the centuries. As well as appealing to these gods for good fortune, people often ask them for protection against evil.

Feng shui (wind and water) is another popular practice involving the placing of objects in the home in a way that will be in harmony with the earth's natural forces (*ch'i*). Correct placement ensures the balance of *yin* and *yang*.

Chinese funerals are associated with elaborate ritual and ceremony, due to the belief that burial without proper ceremony can result in the person not finding their way to Heaven but remaining as a ghost. Before the soul of the deceased can ascend to heaven, it must descend to the underworld and explain its actions during life. Good behaviour ensures a faster passage to heaven. The relatives may offer ritual sacrifices to the gods or build model cars or aeroplanes to ensure transport to Heaven.

Christian Science

> Christian Science explains all cause and effect as mental, not physical.
>
> Mary Baker Eddy, *Science and Health with Key to the Scriptures*

Origin

Christian Science started in Boston in 1879. There are no ordained clergy, but there are teachers, readers and healing practitioners. These practitioners will offer prayer for the patient, and their contact details can be found in the *Christian Science Journal.*

Books and writings

The most widely read book is *Science and Health with Key to the Scriptures* by Mary Baker Eddy, published in 1875. Mrs Eddy claimed that this book was a revelation from God.

Christian Scientists might ask for a *Bible*, but will also wish to read *Science and Health with Key to the Scriptures* or their own daily newspaper (*Christian Science Journal*), which may be obtained from the Christian Science Reading Room that is maintained by each Christian Scientist Church.

Summary of teachings

God is not a person, nor is God triune. God is referred to as 'Life', 'Truth' or 'Mind'.

Mankind was created perfect and never departed from that state. Therefore there is no need for forgiveness. There is no eternal punishment. Because God is everything, Satan does not exist, nor does evil exist except in one's mind.

Christian Scientists dispute the reality of sickness and death. Suffering, sickness and pain are all in our mind and do not actually exist. Disease can be overcome by prayer alone. They believe that the healing miracles of Jesus recorded in the *Bible* are the outcome of understanding the spiritual law that is available in every age.

Christian Scientists believe that because there is no such thing as evil, there is neither a Hell nor punishment for unforgiven sin after death. Punishment for sin lasts for as long as we believe in it, because it only exists in our mortal minds. A terminal illness should therefore hold no fear in this respect for the Christian Scientist.

Beliefs and traditions with regard to illness

Christian Scientists believe that, because physical illness does not exist, drug treatment is not necessary. They will accept setting of fractures and surgical treatment, and some may accept analgesia for severe pain. Transplants are not normally acceptable.

Since blood transfusion is a 'material' method of treatment, it may be refused, as their desire is to rely only on spiritual means of healing.

Terminal illness and death

There are no special requirements as the time of death approaches, except that patients would usually wish a fellow Christian Scientist to be there to support them and their family members.

Christian Scientists do not celebrate Holy Communion with the use of bread and wine, so this sacrament should not be offered.

Transplants and organ donation are not accepted, as these violate the body. Similarly, the use of the body for medical research is seen as a violation.

Euthanasia and physician-assisted suicide are strongly opposed, as no case is believed to be beyond the healing power of God.

It is preferable but not essential that, after death, a female body is handled by female staff. Cremation is usual, but this is a matter for the family to decide.

Hinduism

Origin

The word 'Hindu' originates from the word *Sindhu*, which refers to the Indus river to the north west of India in Pakistan. A flowing river is seen as a living symbol of ongoing life, just as the river flows into the sea and falls as rain replenishing the rivers.

Hinduism is a mixture of religious beliefs and ceremonies that have been practised for some 4500 years in India, but there is no specific recorded date for its origins.

Hinduism has no single founder or prophet, but rather it is a way of life that attempts to free its followers from worldly cares so that they can appreciate what is true and eternal.

The way in which Hinduism is practised varies from region to region.

Books and writings

The earliest writings are a collection of four texts called the *Vedas* which were written around 1000 BC. Much later on, the *Upanishads* appeared. These are a collection of philosophical writings that provide answers to life's questions about our origin and what happens when we die.

The Hindu teaching divides life into four parts:

1 Brahmacharya – the time of education
2 Garhasthya – the time of working
3 Vanapastha – the time of retreating and loosening worldly ties
4 Pravrajya – the time of awaiting freedom through death.

Hindus believe in a return to earth in a form that may be better or worse according to one's '*karma*'. The doctrine of '*karma*' teaches that what an individual does in this world affects what happens to them in the next. Good health is regarded by some as the reward for adhering closely to the religious and moral laws. Hindus believe that one is born to experience the results of past lives, to die again and eventually to be liberated. There are several states of liberation which are not clearly defined, but the highest is to serve Vishnu (the preserver) or Shiva (the destroyer and regenerator of life).

Summary of teachings

Hinduism has thousands of gods and goddesses, although most Hindus insist that these are different manifestations of one God. Among the innumerable other gods there are three supreme gods – Brahma (the creator), Vishnu (the preserver) and Shiva (the destroyer and regenerator of life). These three form the Hindu Trinity. Within Hinduism there are various sects with quite different philosophies and principally worshipping one of the three supreme gods.

Worship can take place in various ways, ranging from quiet meditation to twice-daily temple visits.

Hindus believe in reincarnation, so that they are reborn into the world, their new identity being dictated by their behaviour in their previous life. The ultimate goal is to achieve *moksha* – deliverance from time into eternity *(Brahman)* – the source and origin of creation.

Beliefs and traditions with regard to illness

Hindus have a well-defined philosophy, the *Ayurveda*, which advocates a carefully planned routine of sleep, diet, personal hygiene and physical exercise in moderation.

Some Hindus may regard their final illness as the result of some breach of this code of conduct, and may feel guilt. In the western world there may be some conflict between the teachings and theories of modern medicine and the teachings of Ayurveda. A Hindu priest should be asked to give advice if this is causing the patient anxiety.

Washing is an important aspect of Hindu life. This includes washing the hands and rinsing the mouth before and after eating.

Fasting on a regular basis is common, and this may cause concern with regard to adequate fluid intake. Prolonged fasting may have implications for medications that should be taken after food to reduce the risk of irritation to the stomach lining. Although one can advise, the final decision about fasting rests with the patient.

Personal care, including help with washing and dressing, should be provided by a carer of the same sex. Hindus will not normally discuss any problems or discomfort relating to their bowel or urinary function, so constipation associated with morphine and similar painkillers may go unreported.

Terminal illness and death

Hindus believe that the body should be kept pure, as should the mind. A daily bath in running water (e.g. a shower) is the preferred method of cleansing, preferably first thing in the morning, before praying. Because Hindu teaching includes the belief that bathing renders one spiritually clean, the daily washing routine may be of particular importance to a terminally ill Hindu patient.

Most Hindus regard death as of little significance, because they believe that they will be at one with God in their life after death. A person's death is followed by rebirth, with the birth and death cycle continuing until they are liberated. Exactly what is believed to happen after death varies from one Hindu tradition to another. Several types of temporary paradise (svarga) are described, as well as several types of Hell. Each action in life earns either merit or demerit. The balance determines one's next existence.

As death approaches, the Hindu patient will be helped by the presence of a priest (pandit) who can assist with personal acts of worship and preparation for death, which is usually accepted philosophically, in keeping with Hindu teachings.

After death, the body may be placed on the floor (customs vary) and incense may be burned. There is no restriction on who handles the body, but post-mortem examinations are strongly resisted. Cremation is the normal practice, and the ashes are usually scattered over water in a river or lake. Water from the river Ganges may be brought to the funeral, and in some cases the family may wish to consult with the funeral director for transportation of the body to be cremated by the river Ganges.

Further reading on Hinduism

- Narayanan V. *Understanding Hindusm.* London: Duncan Baird Publishers; 2004.

Humanism

Origin

Humanism is not a religion, but is included here in case you need to know more about the patient's humanist beliefs, as these could affect how they wish to be treated at the end of life.

Humanism arose as a movement in the fourteenth century in Italy. Humanism was the essence of the Renaissance, and involved a revival of study of the works of the Latin and Greek philosophers, searching for what they actually meant without a specifically Christian interpretation of their writings.

Protagoras (*c*.450 BC) wrote that 'Man is the measure of all things. As for the gods, I do not know whether they exist or not. Life is too short for such difficult enquiries.'

Epicures (342–270 BC) summed up the views that were becoming accepted by a small but growing minority when he wrote, 'Become accustomed to the belief that death is nothing to us. For all good and evil consist in sensation, but death is the deprivation of sensation and therefore a right understanding that death is nothing makes life enjoyable.'

Humanism became a point of view, asserting human dignity and values and expressing a confidence in the ability of humanity to exert control over nature and to shape society according to the needs of the people.

Modern humanism is defined as 'a philosophy that puts the emphasis on humans solving the problems of life without the dogmatic authority of secular or religious institutions'.

Summary of teachings

Humanists were tolerant of all religious viewpoints, regarding the diversity of denominations and religions as different ways of expressing one truth. The Church was not so tolerant of this viewpoint, since it challenged the teachings of the *Bible*, and centuries of conflict followed. By the seventeenth and eighteenth centuries, an intellectual movement known as 'the Enlightenment' had been formed, which had its roots firmly in humanism.

The Enlightenment movement had the aim of understanding the natural world and humankind's place in it solely on the basis of reason and without turning to religious belief. Most Enlightenment thinkers did not reject religion completely, but accepted the existence of God and a hereafter, while rejecting the Christian theology of creation, sin and divine damnation.

Modern humanism also embraces the following teachings.

- Rational thought and responsible behaviour will enhance quality of life on earth.
- Humans exist along with other life forms, and nature is indifferent to our individual existence.
- The meaning and purpose of life must be found in living, not dying.
- Moral values are not divinely revealed, nor are they the special property of any religious tradition. They must be found by humans by use of natural reasoning, and our belief in what is right or wrong must be constantly subjected to the deepest reflection in the light of our evolving understanding of our nature and our world.
- *Humanists have faith in the human capacity to choose good over evil, but without the expectation of any reward in another life.*

Beliefs and traditions with regard to illness

In terms of palliative care and the issues concerning advance directives (living wills), Dr James Fletcher, who was voted 'Humanist of the Year' in 1974, said 'We should drop the sanctity-of-life ethic and embrace a quality-of-life ethic'.

Humanists will accept treatment, but may ask for consideration of an advance directive.

Terminal illness and death

Humanists do not believe in a God who is involved in human behaviour or way of life. The funeral is therefore a celebration of the life lived and an opportunity to encourage support for the bereaved.

Further information may be obtained from the British Humanist Association, London. (Tel: 020 7079 3580.)

Further reading on humanism

- *Compton's Interactive Encyclopedia. Enlightenment.* The Learning Company, Inc.; 1999.
- *Compton's Interactive Encyclopedia. Humanism.* The Learning Company, Inc.; 1999.
- Gilmore MP. *The World of Humanism, 1453–1517.* London: Harper & Row; 1962.
- Wineriter F. *Living and Dying: humanism, a rational approach to life and death.* Text of a lecture presented on 14 September 2000.

Islam

Origin

Islam is the religion practised by Muslims, and is based on the writings of Muhammad, who lived around 1400 years ago. Islam is a whole way of life with legal, moral, political and spiritual guidelines, so that every action and thought is guided by complete submission to Allah.

Books and writings

Islam literally means 'submission to God', and is practised by Muslim patients. Islam is based on the teachings of the prophet Muhammad, whom Muslims believe to have received the final revealed word of Allah. Muslims believe that some parts of the divine teachings were revealed in the past through other prophets, including Moses and Jesus Christ, and this final message from Allah is contained in the *Koran (Qur'an)*, which cannot be altered or added to.

Summary of teachings

There are five 'Pillars of Islam' that support the beliefs and practices of the Islamic faith. These can be summarised as follows.

1 Shahada – the statement of faith, which includes the statement 'I bear witness that there is no God but Allah, and I bear witness that Muhammad is the messenger of Allah'.
2 Salat – daily worship. Prayers are recited at dawn, midday, in the afternoon, in the evening and at night, bowing low down in the direction of Mecca (south-east in the UK). The exact times of sunrise and sunset are used to determine the prayer times. Before praying, one must wash the face, ears, forehead, feet, hands and arms to the elbows. The nose is cleaned by sniffing water and the mouth is rinsed.
3 Zakat – charitable giving, which copies the generosity of Allah, partly atones for one's sins and shows practical kindness to the less well off.

4 Sawm – fasting, which involves going without food and drink during the hours of daylight in the holy month of Ramadan.
5 Hajj – the pilgrimage to Mecca, the birthplace of Muhammad, which healthy Muslim men and women are expected to make at least once in their lifetime.

Islam is a complete way of life, and every action and thought should be guided by complete submission to Allah. Friday is the holy day when Muslims visit the mosque.

There is no priest, but the patient might ask for an imam – a learned man of the Muslim faith – to visit. The nearest Islamic centre should be contacted, details of which should be available in the telephone directory.

Beliefs and traditions with regard to illness

Muslims do not eat any form of meat that is of porcine origin, and this includes anything cooked in pig fat. Failure to wash utensils after using them to serve pork renders the food they touch unclean. Meat should be killed according to Muslim law. Some patients might find it preferable for their food to be specially prepared and brought in for them.

The patient will wish to wash five times a day before prayer, and will need to know the direction of Mecca.

Technically, the acutely ill and chronically sick have the option of not fasting during Ramadan, but may be reluctant to do this. The Quran specifically exempts the sick from the duty of fasting if the latter may lead to harmful consequences for an individual (*Qur'an* 2: 183–185). If the long hours of daylight in the northern hemisphere cause problems (e.g. for diabetics), the local imam should be contacted so that he can discuss the problem with the patient (and her husband, if the patient is a woman).

Drugs and alcohol are expressly forbidden, but allowance may be made for drugs being used for medical purposes. However, porcine insulin and other pig products are still forbidden.

Pain is usually seen as the will of Allah, and his will should not be resisted. Patients might wish to have the support of relatives and friends from the local Islamic centre if they feel unable to accept analgesia.

Modesty is of great importance. Women find contact with a male member of staff humiliating, and it renders them unclean. Men are dubious about being treated by women, and may think of them as of low status for having physical contact with a 'strange man'. Dress is also important, and the dress code should be respected.

Muslims have very strong feelings about graft and transplant surgery. Muslims may not receive a transplant, nor can they donate their organs, even among members of their own faith. Tissue grafts of porcine origin are also forbidden.

Terminal illness and death

The Islamic tradition maintains that there is an afterlife, and more may be learned about this from the *Koran*, the *Hadith* (the record of Muhammed's life) and the other sacred literature.

For the terminally ill Muslim, Ramadan is the final opportunity to put their personal spiritual affairs in order. Fasting includes not ingesting anything by mouth, nose, suppository or injection, from dawn to sunset. This may cause problems with symptom control, but many patients will derive comfort from being able to comply with their religious laws. The use of analgesics with a 24-hour action, offered at a suitable time of day, might represent an acceptable form of pain relief.

Special prayers are recited in Arabic, regardless of nationality. If possible, the patient should join in, facing Mecca. Relatives or Muslims from the local mosque might also wish to recite prayers. The last words that a Muslim should utter (always facing Mecca) are the *shahada* – the first words spoken to them at birth – *'There is no God but Allah, and Muhammad is his prophet'*. Muslims believe that after death, which is seen as a transformation into a new phase of existence, Allah will judge their good and bad deeds, including their charitable giving, and their final utterance of the *shahada* in the hope of mercy in the afterlife.

Death is the decision by God to end a person's physical life on earth. It is a shift from one mode of life to another. Death is not regarded as permanent – the physical body decays, but the soul (*nafs*) moves on to a new plane. The *Koran* speaks of heaven and hell, describing Heaven as a place of beauty where 'rivers flow' (*Sura* 98, 9), and describing Hell as 'a fire burning fiercely' (*Sura* 1018, 11).

After death it is preferred that only Muslims should touch the body. If this is not possible, disposable gloves must be worn and the family should be consulted before any procedure is carried out. The body should be wrapped in a sheet and be positioned with the face pointing towards Mecca. The body will later be washed according to Islamic tradition and wrapped in cloth. Men are wrapped in three pieces of cloth, and women are wrapped in five pieces. Men must not see or touch a female body after death. Coffins are not acceptable, nor is autopsy. If an autopsy is suggested, the reasons for it being carried out must be discussed with the family.

It is important that burial should take place as quickly as possible, usually the morning after death. A member of the Muslim community, who will advise the undertaker of the strict code of practice that is followed, usually arranges the funeral. Embalming is not usually carried out, and in the UK the body is usually buried, wrapped in a sheet, without a coffin. A coffin may be used for transportation only.

The orientation of the grave is very important, as the body must be placed with the face turned towards Mecca. The surface of the grave must be raised above ground level (which contravenes some cemetery by-laws), so a special area may be set aside for Muslim burials.

Further information may be found at www.IslamReligion.com.

Further reading on Islam

- Aadil N, Houti IE, Moussamih S. Drug intake during Ramadan. *BMJ.* 2004; **329:** 788–9.
- Gordon MS. *Understanding Islam.* London: Duncan Baird Publishers; 2002.
- Sarhill N, Mahmoud F, Walsh D. Muslim beliefs regarding death and bereavement. *Eur J Palliat Care.* 2003; **10:** 34–7.
- Sheikh A, Gatrad AR. *Caring for Muslim Patients.* Oxford: Radcliffe Medical Press; 2000.

Jehovah's Witnesses

Summary of teachings

In a hospital or hospice setting, Jehovah's Witnesses do not have any special requirements with regard to how they are cared for and treated. Their refusal of blood does not include food (except black pudding), as modern slaughter methods are deemed adequate for the removal of unwanted blood.

The real issue is that of blood transfusions. Most Jehovah's Witnesses will either be carrying a card or will happily sign the standard form used by most hospitals. This releases you from responsibility for the outcome of such a refusal. The card carried by some Witnesses directs that no blood should be given, and is signed by the patient and two witnesses, of whom one is usually a family member and the other a congregation elder or a solicitor, both of whom are authorised to uphold this decision in the event that the patient cannot express their own wishes.

As new artificial blood products become available, the Watchtower Society, which is the authoritative body governing the Jehovah's Witnesses movement, has issued new guidance, and this has been updated and may change as new instructions are issued by the Watchtower Society.

Strictly speaking, it is only baptised Witnesses who must refuse blood transfusions, and no sanctions can be taken against a person who is not a baptised member and who has accepted a blood transfusion. However, it is important to recognise that many non-baptised Witnesses will refuse transfusions, and parents of children may refuse due to their duty to 'bring up their children in the training and instruction of the Lord' (as instructed in Ephesians 6:4, New International Version of the *Bible*).

You are advised to ask the patient or an elder from the local Kingdom Hall for current advice if the situation is unclear.

Taking blood samples for investigations is acceptable, and most treatments are accepted.

Terminal illness and death

A dying Jehovah's Witness will wish to be visited by friends and family and elders from their local Kingdom Hall. There are no clergy as such, since all Witnesses are ministers to each other, so the congregation will expect the same visiting privileges as a minister from another faith.

There are no ceremonial rites at death, there is no objection to a post-mortem, and the use of the body for medical research is a matter of individual decision. Burial and cremation are equally acceptable.

Organ transplantation is unlikely to be an issue in cancer patients, but corneas may be acceptable, as there is no blood involved.

All forms of hastening death – by euthanasia, physician-assisted suicide or abortion – are strongly opposed, but striving to prolong life unnecessarily is not expected.

Medical staff may wish to address specific queries to the Medical Desk, The Watchtower Bible and Tract Society, Watchtower House, The Ridgeway, London NW7 1RN. (No direct telephone number or email address was available.)

Judaism

Origin

Judaism is the world's oldest monotheistic religion – one that accepts that there is one God, who created the world and continues to rule over it.

Books and writings

The word of God was revealed to Moses around 3,500 years ago in the Ten Commandments. The first five books of the Old Testament of the Bible are also known as the Torah.

Summary of teachings

Judaism has the central belief that everything is under the control of God. God created man, and man's purpose is to recognise and serve God, to live a just life, to perform good deeds, to study the Torah and to live accordingly.

The Torah is sometimes referred to as the Written Law, but in addition to this there is the Oral Law contained in the Talmud, the body of Jewish civil and ceremonial law and legend comprising the Mishnah and the Gemara, written between the third and sixth centuries.

Judiasm is therefore sometimes described as a way of life rather than a religion, since it is very much concerned with keeping the Jewish law.

The Jews do not venerate Jesus or believe that He is God's Messiah, nor do they celebrate Christmas or Easter, since these Christian festivals celebrate the birth, death and resurrection of Jesus as the Son of God.

The Sabbath (which lasts from sundown on Friday to sundown on Saturday) is a very important day for the religious Jew, and New Year, the festival of the Passover and the Day of Atonement are also very important days to be observed. To a varying degree, Jews keep the law as laid down in the Ten Commandments.

Although Jews believe that the soul is immortal, they concentrate much more on practical issues that make this world a better place in which to live.

Beliefs and traditions with regard to illness

Even the most non-religious Jew retains a very strong sense of the value of human life on the basis that God created man in His own image (Genesis 1: 27). This belief in preservation of life is so strong that one may even break certain religious laws in order to preserve a human life. In practice, this means that the terminally ill Jew need not observe festivals or the Sabbath, although many will choose to do so.

An ill Jew will appreciate the lighting of a candle at the beginning of the Sabbath, and will also appreciate being given unleavened bread at Passover. (Unleavened bread is relatively easily obtained.) In addition, a visit from a Rabbi at Passover will be greatly appreciated.

There are several laws relating to food, the main ones being the forbidding of pork and shellfish, and the avoidance of serving meat and milk in the same meal. (This practice relates to the instruction in Exodus 23:19 – 'Do not cook a young goat in its mother's milk.') An interval of 6 hours between consuming meat and drinking milk is usually acceptable.

Terminal illness and death

Food is very important in Jewish life, and the family of a terminally ill Jew might bring in food to try to tempt the patient to eat. To the non-Jew, this concern about food may seem inappropriate, but in Judaism, it is this life that matters and eating is a sign of holding on to this life and staying in this world. Orthodox Jews do believe in the resurrection of the dead and an afterlife, but the details of what they actually believe vary widely from one person to another.

The importance of the 'here and now' can cause problems for the Jew when dealing with dying patients. Someone who is dying – who will not be in this world for much longer – is not seen as being as important as someone who has a longer life to anticipate. Any form of euthanasia or attempt to shorten life is strongly resisted.

As death approaches, Jews are encouraged to confess their sins to the Great Judge, indicating a belief in the continuing existence of the soul, although Judaism is vague on this area of its teaching. It is desirable to die uttering the *Shema*, Judaism's central confession of faith in one indivisible God, based on the words of Deuteronomy 6:4–9, quoted here from the New International Version of the *Bible*:

> 4: Hear, O Israel: The Lord our God, the Lord is one.
> 5: Love the Lord your God with all your heart and with all your soul and with all your strength.
> 6: These commandments that I give you today are to be upon your hearts.
> 7: Impress them on your children. Talk about them when you sit at home and when you walk along the road, when you lie down and when you get up.
> 8: Tie them as symbols on your hands and bind them on your foreheads.
> 9: Write them on the door-frames of your houses and on your gates.

A dying Jew might ask to see the Rabbi. There are no last rites, so a visit is not essential, but if the patient does ask to see the Rabbi, find out whether they are an orthodox or non-orthodox Jew and which Rabbi should be called.

After death, it is traditional for the body to be placed on the floor, with the feet pointing towards the door and a burning candle placed near the head. Fellow Jews or family members usually take responsibility for the care of the body, with someone watching over it day and night, reciting psalms continually. This period of watching is not very long, as burial should take place as quickly as possible.

Orthodox Jews are buried in a Jewish cemetery within 24 hours of the death. More liberal Jews may allow cremation, and the family usually arranges the funeral, which may take place 2 or 3 days after the death.

A period of mourning then takes place, initially for 7 days, but the full period of mourning is 30 days, and after one year the tombstone is consecrated, marking the end of formal mourning.

In the orthodox Jewish religion, post-mortem examinations are resisted and the donation of organs for transplant is not encouraged. The traditional view is that, since man was created in God's image, it is abhorrent to mutilate the body in this way. A post-mortem will usually only be accepted if required by law.

Some more liberal Jews are more relaxed about these laws, so it is worth finding out the family's wishes.

Further reading

- Ehrlich CS. *Understanding Judaism.* London: Duncan Baird Publishers; 2004.
- Neuberger J. Judaism and palliative care. *Eur J Palliat Care.* 1999; **6:** 166–8.
- Spitzer J. *Caring for Jewish Patients.* Oxford: Radcliffe Medical Press; 2003.

Mormonism

The members of the Church of Jesus Christ of Latter Day Saints are also known as Mormons.

Books and writings

The *Book of Mormon* is regarded as an addition to the *Bible*, and is central to the beliefs of the Church of Jesus Christ of Latter Day Saints.

Summary of teachings

There is a belief in pre-existence in a spirit world prior to physical birth, but due to the erasure of all memory of the spiritual world, the newborn infant has no recollection of their previous existence. After death, the spirit leaves the body, returns to the spiritual place and eventually body and spirit are reunited in resurrection. Life on this earth thus determines one's status in the next. Antecedents who have died but who were not members of the Church of Jesus Christ of Latter Day Saints may be baptised into the church and 'sealed' with their families for eternity. Death is therefore regarded with only a temporary sadness.

Children under the age of 8 years are deemed not to have reached the 'age of accountability', and thus are incapable of sin. There is therefore no requirement for the emergency baptism of a young child who is dying.

Mormons abstain from alcohol, so if one is preparing for the sacrament of Holy Communion, the elements used are bread and water, not bread and wine.

Terminal illness and death

Mormons eat meat sparingly, and avoid eating black pudding and receiving blood products, but do accept blood transfusions. All stimulants, including tea, coffee and alcohol, are forbidden. Some Mormons refuse all hot drinks.

Spiritual contact is important, and the Mormon patient will usually know which Bishop should be contacted. 'Home Teachers' will visit either home or hospital and look after various needs.

Members of the Melchizedek Priesthood may give a 'priesthood blessing', but otherwise there are no special rituals or preparations.

Some Mormons, who have been through a special Temple ceremony, wear a special undergarment which is worn in health, illness and death. It is an intensely personal item, must not be exposed to public display and must be treated with respect. After death, this garment must be placed on the body after the routine last offices have been carried out.

Transplants are a matter for decision by the individual. Post-mortems are acceptable, and there is no teaching about the avoidance of donation of the body to medical research.

All forms of euthanasia, physician-assisted suicide and abortion are opposed. Burial is preferred and cremation is not encouraged.

Sikhism

Origin

The term 'Sikh' means 'follower', and the Sikh religion was founded in the fifteenth century by Guru Nanak (1469–1533). ('Guru' means spiritual guide.) Sikhism had its origins in the Punjab when Guru Nanak was examining the differences between Hinduism and Islam. Being unsure which path to follow, he founded a new religion – Sikhism.

The Sikh religion has a strong community aspect, and the Sikh temple (gurdwara) is a place of gathering and group activity.

There is no priesthood among Sikhs, with each gurdwara providing the services required in their local Sikh community. Births, marriages, etc. are all celebrated in the gurdwara.

Books and writings

Sikhism has 10 Gurus, and their collective writings are contained in the *Guru Granth Sahib*. This book is the basis of all Sikh ceremonies and is written in Punjabi. All Sikhs learn to read the Guru Granth Sahib.

Summary of teachings

God created the world and everything in it, but because He is not visible in creation, His will must be made known through the Gurus.

Sikhism is associated with five symbols of faith – known as 'the five Ks'.

- *Kesh* – uncut hair covered by a turban. The hair is kept in a bun (jura) by both men and women. Women don't usually wear a turban, but men do.
- *Kanga* – the comb, symbolising personal hygiene. A small semi-circular comb is used by both men and women to keep the bun in position. The kanga is a very significant item to a Sikh, and if it cannot be in their hair (e.g. if the patient has lost their hair due to chemotherapy), they will want it to be close by, and it should never be removed or tidied away.
- *Kara* – the steel bracelet representing faithfulness to God (originally a protection for the arm carrying the sword). The circular shape represents the unity of God. It should never be removed.
- *Kirpan* – the dagger, symbolising resistance to evil and the Sikh's readiness to fight in self-defence and to protect the poor and oppressed. The size, shape and position of the kirpan and where it is worn all vary. It is important to recognise that the kirpan is worn all the time – at night, in the shower, and so on. Do not attempt to remove it on the grounds that it may cause injury while the patient is sleeping – this causes great distress and may result in the patient losing trust in you and failing to seek help when necessary. If removal is absolutely necessary, the reasons must be fully discussed with the patient and their family, and the kirpan must be kept within sight of the patient.
- *Kaccha* – special shorts (underpants), symbolising purity. Traditionally kaccha were knee length, but many Sikhs now wear ordinary underpants instead. As a symbol of modesty and sexual morality, their removal may be strongly resisted. It is common practice for them to be worn in the shower, with a dry pair replacing the wet ones afterwards. During practical procedures such as

bed-bathing, one leg should always be kept in the kaccha. This is especially important in dying patients.

Beliefs and traditions with regard to illness

Because the gurdwara is the focal point of all activity, any illness that prevents attendance at the gurdwara causes considerable distress. It is common for the gurdwara to arrange for someone to visit and sit with a dying patient.

Traditionally Sikhs rise very early to allow time to wash and spend about 2 hours in prayer before breakfast. Illness may make this difficult, so the offer of help with washing before prayer will be appreciated. During prayer one should respect the Sikh's privacy, and they will be appreciate being left alone.

Terminal illness and death

Sikhs believe that the soul goes through multiple cycles of birth and rebirth, so dying is not frightening. The ultimate aim is to achieve perfection and be reunited with God. How one behaves in this life affects their next life. Fear of dying is therefore likely to be associated with anxiety about what their next life will be like.

After death, the family is usually responsible for looking after the body. Cremation is usual, with the 'five Ks' being worn on the body. If possible, the cremation should take place within 24 hours of the death. The ashes are usually scattered in a river or the sea.

After the cremation, family and friends will gather at the gurdwara for further prayers before returning home, where it is usual for them to have a shower. The period of mourning lasts for 10–13 days, during which time relatives and friends visit to comfort the bereaved. The home might be used as a temporary temple, with furniture being removed, the floor covered and a canopy erected. If this is not possible, the gurdwara can be used.

At the end of the period of mourning, if the deceased was the head of the family, another ceremony takes place to acknowledge the eldest son as head of the family. A lamp may be kept lit for several weeks in memory of the deceased person.

Further reading about spiritual and religious issues with regard to illness

- Barnes T. *The Kingfisher Book of Religions.* London: Kingfisher Publications plc; 1999.
- Biechele I, Roser T. Why palliative care cannot exist without spiritual care. *Eur J Palliat Care.* 2005; **12:** 263–4.
- Green J, Green M. *Dealing with Death.* London: Chapman and Hall; 1992.
- Helman C. *Culture, Health and Illness.* London: Butterworth-Heinemann; 2000.
- Murray S, Kendall M, Boyd K *et al.* General practitioners and their possible role in providing spiritual care: a qualitative study. *Br J Gen Pract.* 2003; **53:** 957–9.
- Neuberger J. *Caring for Dying People of Different Faiths.* Oxford: Radcliffe Publishing; 2004.
- Neuberger J. *Dying Well.* Oxford: Radcliffe Publishing; 2004.
- Reoch R. *Dying Well.* London: Gaia Books Ltd; 1997.
- Sampson C. *The Neglected Ethic: cultural and religious factors in the care of patients.* London: McGraw-Hill; 1982.
- Scaon S, Chasseigne G, Colombat P. Perception of the spiritual needs of patients. *Eur J Palliat Care.* 2006; **13:** 39–40.
- Sheikh A, Gatrad AR. *Caring for Muslim Patients.* Oxford: Radcliffe Medical Press; 2000.
- Spiro H, Curnen MG, Wandel LP. *Facing Death.* London: Yale University Press; 1996.
- Spitzer J. *Caring for Jewish Patients.* Oxford: Radcliffe Medical Press; 2003.

Part 7

Quick practical guides

Anger and aggression: management

Aggression towards staff is becoming more common, and is something that we all have to deal with at some point. Substance abuse or personality disorders may be responsible, but in a palliative care setting, it often arises from perceived delays in diagnosis or from anger and frustration associated with the recognition that one has been robbed of the opportunity to achieve certain goals, or robbed of life itself.

Common causes of anger

- Anxiety and fear.
- Bad news, whether given well or badly.
- Delays (or perceived delays) in getting a diagnosis.
- Delays in being seen.
- Lack of choices.
- Loss of control.
- Personality disorder.
- Substance abuse or withdrawal (including alcohol).

Warning signs

- Verbal – voice slow, soft or loud, or sudden use of abusive language.
- Violent behaviour – getting close, raised arms or other threatening movement.
- Visual – loss of eye contact, frowning, reddening of the face, etc.

Do

- Acknowledge any shortfalls in the system, but explain why the system has 'failed'.
- Acknowledge their reasons for being upset.
- Apologise, if appropriate, but do not take blame unfairly.
- Be assertive but not aggressive in stating the facts honestly.
- Explain the reasons for perceived delays.
- Explore exactly what they think went wrong.
- Keep a safe distance.
- Listen 'actively', with eye contact and appropriate nods and signs of listening.
- Retain your composure.
- Stay calm.

Do not

- Be defensive, making remarks like 'We did our best'.
- Block access to the door.
- Challenge the patient's ability to make a judgement.
- Deny genuine errors or mistakes that have been picked up.
- Get angry (even if your qualifications or experience are questioned).
- Interrupt.
- Speak from behind the patient – make eye contact.
- Touch the patient to pacify them – this may be seen as assault.

'BEFRIENDING' the patient

To give the patient our best care, we need to *befriend them*. The word 'befriend' reminds us to think about the patient's:

- **B**eliefs
- **E**ducation
- **F**amily
- **R**eligion
- **I**nfection risk
- **E**xpectations
- **N**utrition
- **D**ifficulties they are experiencing.

We have included a few examples under each of these headings, and you will be able to add many more of your own.

B Beliefs

- Cultural.
- Personal.
- Religious.

E Education

- About the illness.
- About the treatment.
- About the probable prognosis.

F Family

- Do the values and beliefs of the family conflict with those of the patient?
- Consent – is there agreement about who gives consent to treatment if the patient is under age or has impaired understanding?
- How are other members of the family coping with their relative's illness?

R Religion

- Are there any issues that affect acceptance of treatment (e.g. Jehovah's Witness and blood transfusion)? What about compliance with medications during Ramadan, when the patient cannot eat or drink anything (including medications) from dawn to sunset?
- Do the patient's religious beliefs affect how they view their illness in terms of acceptance of the illness, prognosis and/or treatment?

I Infection risk

- Has fear of picking up an infection resulted in the patient not receiving appropriate care from the family or other carers?

E Expectations

- Are the patient's past experiences affecting their present/future expectations?
- Is the anticipated outcome of the present illness and the future realistic?

N Nutrition

- What are the effects of the illness or treatment on the patient's nutritional state? Is there any loss of appetite?
- Are the patient's cultural dietary needs being met? Is the appropriate ethnic diet available?
- Think about foods, festivals and religious fasts (e.g. Yom Kippur or Ramadan).

D Difficulties they are experiencing

- Difficulty getting to hospital appointments.
- Problems with daily life.
- Unpleasant or painful symptoms and associated problems.
- Communication problems – sensory impairment/speech difficulty.
- Lack of fluency in your language.
- Learning disability.

Clinical audit and clinical effectiveness

In our discussions, there were many comments about the increasing importance of clinical audit and clinical effectiveness. Several interviewees expressed anxiety about these subjects. We offer only the most basic thoughts here, based on teaching notes used by WF for small group work.

To assess how effective our care is, we must conduct regular audits. Auditing our performance can be threatening, but we must focus on the opportunity that it provides to identify areas where care can be improved and ensure that the necessary changes are made, in order to safeguard high standards of care. Does the idea of audit leave you 'hot and bothered'? Try the clinical audit ice cube!

The clinical audit ICE CUBE

- **I**dentify the subject to be audited.
- **C**hoose the standard for comparison.
- **E**vidence for your present performance.
- **C**ompare with the chosen standard.
- **U**nsatisfactory performance? Identify and then
- **B**egin the necessary changes.
- **E**valuate the outcome.

Why does clinical effectiveness MATTER?

- Because one must choose the right **M**ethod
- To carry out the appropriate **A**ctivity
- At the right **T**ime
- Using the proper **T**ools
- In the hands of a person with **E**xpertise
- To offer the best care to the **R**ecipient.

Communicating with deputising staff

Working as the weekend doctor or nurse in the community is challenging when you are called to see a patient you don't know. A brief written case summary is invaluable when one is called out to see a patient whose needs are changing, often on a daily basis.

An outline summary could usefully contain the following information.

Administrative information

- Details of the patient, including hospital reference numbers and the names of the consultants involved in order to facilitate more efficient access to hospital clinical records.
- The names and contact details of the regular GP and other primary care team members.
- Consultant and hospital details, so that the appropriate team can be contacted.

Clinical information

- Diagnosis.
- Summary of recent developments and progress of the illness.
- Relevant recent medical history.
- Current medications, recent changes and instructions given for management of changing symptoms (e.g. breakthrough pain doses, etc.).
- Investigations and blood tests currently awaited, if relevant.

Other relevant information

- Details of the carers, including any private input, Macmillan/Marie Curie services, etc.
- Any booked admissions or other planned appointments that may be relevant or could be speeded up if necessary.

Occasionally one meets patients who are unaware of the truth or unwilling to discuss their situation openly. If this is an issue, be sensitive when writing your notes.

Completing a death certificate

The death certificate:

- allows the relatives to register the death and arrange the funeral
- provides legal evidence concerning a death
- provides mortality statistics for resource allocation in the NHS and for the public health and epidemiological services.

Death certificates can be issued if the doctor:

- has seen the patient within the previous 2 weeks before the death
- is satisfied that the death is due to natural causes
- knows the cause of death with reasonable certainty
- thinks that referral to the coroner is unnecessary.

The Coroner's Reform Bill (April 2006) applies in England and Wales and will allow coroners access to independent medical advice to assist in complex cases. Although this is unlikely to arise in the case of cancer patients, one is reminded of the advice of the General Medical Council, which states that 'you must be honest and trustworthy when writing reports'.

Cases that must be reported to the coroner

These include the following:

- cause of death unknown
- death that may be a suicide
- death that may be due to an accident (whenever it occurred)
- death that may be due to self-neglect or neglect by others
- death that may be related to an abortion
- death that may be related to industrial disease or the deceased's employment
- death that occurred during an operation or before recovery from the effects of an anaesthetic
- death that occurred during or shortly after detention in prison or police custody
- death that was violent, suspicious or unnatural
- deceased not seen by the certifying doctor either after death or within 14 days before death.

Dictating letters

This might seem an unusual topic to include, but since there is a tendency for many doctors to send out letters unsigned and unchecked, it is reasonable to try to get the facts right!

The authors believe that your colleagues deserve to receive a letter which you dictated, checked, confirmed, amended if necessary and signed, but we recognise that we live in the 'real' world, not the 'ideal' one! We are aware that at least one medical newspaper publishes a badly written letter each week. Although we might find them amusing, they represent a failure of communication, due to a simple and avoidable lack of attention to detail.

Planning

If it is a long letter, spend a few minutes planning the content, and include the information necessary to allow the recipient to answer any questions that will arise, recognising that they are dependent on your letter for the necessary information.

Put important information in a summary near the top of the letter.

Who are you writing to?

Before you write, think about what the recipient needs to know. This is not an excuse to leave out less important information, but should help you to prioritise what is most relevant and what should be made easily accessible.

Helping your secretary

Speak clearly, and don't have lunch at the same time! The typist has to cope with your accent, background noise and sometimes unfamiliar words, so be realistic and make life as easy as possible, thereby reducing the opportunity for mistakes.

Spell unfamiliar terms and drug names, especially as some spellings have changed to accommodate the 'rINNs' now used for drugs.

Use the internationally recognised phonetic alphabet for letters (e.g. alpha for 'A', and so on).

When using numbers, make sure that numbers ending in '-ty' or '-teen' are identified. For example, if 'forty' is repeated as 'four, zero' and 'fourteen' is repeated as 'one, four', there should be less risk of a mistake. This is very important when including drug doses, especially opioid doses which are not necessarily being given in tablets of standardised prepared strengths.

What to include in a letter

What needs to be said depends on who is writing and to whom. The construction of a letter can make a huge difference, and a simple layout that makes relevant information easily noticed by the recipient is always helpful.

Essentially we can consider two basic scenarios:

- GP referring to a secondary service
- secondary care service replying to the GP.

GP referring to a secondary service

These letters should include the following:

- administrative content, including the patient's details
- clinical content
- psychosocial content.

Administrative content

- Referring GP's name, address, phone number/fax number/email address, and name of regular GP if different.
- Patient's name, address, date of birth, telephone number and next of kin/carer details.
- Date of referral.

Clinical content

- Brief reason for the referral.
- Current medical problems.
- History of presenting problem or complaint and important past medical history.
- Findings on examination.
- Findings on laboratory tests, and details of any test results awaited (and from which laboratory).
- Medications and recent changes, and the outcomes of these changes.
- Medication allergies and adverse reactions.

Psychosocial content

- Social and family history relevant to future care at home.
- What the patient thinks the referral is meant to achieve, and their views about being referred.
- What the relatives think the referral is meant to achieve, and their views about the patient being referred.
- What the GP hopes the referral will achieve, and how they feel care can be managed at home in the future.

Secondary care service replying to GP

- Confirm the history and highlight any differences between what the patient and the referring GP reported when giving the medical history.
- Findings on examination.
- Findings on investigation.
- Problem summary.
- Suggested plan of management.
- What the patient has been told and what he or she expects to happen next.
- What the relatives have been told and what they expect to happen next.
- When, and to whose care, the patient was or will be discharged.
- Who is responsible for following up the patient and when.

Discharge prescriptions

These are sometimes referred to as 'to take out' (TTO) or 'to take away' (TTA).

The handwritten discharge letter and prescription is an important document, but we all know that it is yet another thing to do, and is often asked for at the most inopportune moment! However, it is the working copy for the GP until the full letter eventually reaches the primary care team, so it is a very important document.

What follows is simply common sense, but we include it because our experience is that sometimes these simple rules are not followed, and this can lead to avoidable problems.

Think about the following.

Accuracy and legibility

The discharge letter and prescription is useless if it is incorrect, is open to misinterpretation or can't be read! Use labels with patient details, as they are quick and legible and should be accurate.

Caring team details

Details of the consultant, ward and other agencies/staff involved, with contact details, should be included.

Clinical details

Presenting problems, examinations, investigations, diagnosis, procedures and treatment should all be briefly outlined. This will be the only communication between professional carers until the full letter arrives. Don't put your GP colleague at a disadvantage and the patient at risk for the sake of a few words.

Note: Make sure that any changes to pre-admission drugs are clearly documented. It is far too easy to re-run the original computer-stored prescription printout these days!

Discharge date and place, and to whose care

This information should have been discussed with the GP and all arrangements should be in place, but we do live in the real world, and it is therefore best to include these details for appropriate follow-up action.

Follow-up

Outpatient appointments, tests and investigations, further treatment sessions, etc., should be briefly noted.

Future care

What is the plan? Is the patient likely to be moving to the increasing input and care of another team (e.g. palliative care)?

Readmission

Is readmission to your unit appropriate? If not, where will the patient be best cared for?

Treatments (and any changes to pre-admission drugs)

Write drug names and doses legibly and accurately, and use the generic name or rINN, highlighting changes in dosing schedules for all medications prescribed prior to admission. It is easy to fail to spot a change and re-run the original stored prescription.

Up to date

Here we state the obvious. Don't write the letter in advance. Things can change very rapidly!

End-of-life decisions

There is no simple or solitary formula for end-of-life decision making. The patient's interests come first. We offer a few prompts for you to think through in more detail.

Advance directives

This is a developing and changing area even as we write. Make sure that you are aware of the current law and provision in your area of practice. Where valid, legal and appropriate, the competent patient's advance directive requests must be followed.

Competency

Competency assessment will be required. Make sure that you know what to assess and how it is done. Patients with capacity have the right to refuse or withdraw consent to treatment.

Defence organisation

In the current legal climate, some acts are illegal. Consult your defence organisation before becoming involved in any decision-making process.

Discussion topics

These will almost certainly be of two basic types, and will be about one of two things.

1. *Withholding or withdrawing treatment.* Treatment must confer more benefit than harm or burden. Most of the discussions will be on this topic.
2. *Euthanasia or physician-assisted suicide.* This is a changing area. Be aware of the current law in your area.

DNAR orders

Make every attempt to introduce and discuss the issue of 'Do Not Attempt Resuscitation' orders sensitively and as early as possible. You are not refusing necessary or life-enhancing treatment, but you do need to make a balanced decision as to whether a patient who is dying of cancer wishes to be resuscitated after a cardiopulmonary event.

Family

To avoid misunderstandings, involve the family, with the knowledge and consent of the patient. They may have a valuable point of view that you need to consider. They are the people who have to continue to live with the decision that was taken, so they have a right to be involved and to provide input into the discussion.

GP

The GP should be involved. Their knowledge of the patient is usually much more extensive than yours.

Proxy decision maker

The patient may have appointed an attorney or some other person to make decisions on their behalf. Find out if this is the case, and if it is, consult this person.

Team members

These are not single-person decisions. A team approach that recognises the value of the opinions of senior colleagues is essential.

Witnesses

The opportunity for misunderstood or misreported discussions is obvious. Do not have one-to-one discussions, however simple and unambiguous they may appear.

Write good notes

We feel that we hardly need to say this, but accurate, detailed, signed, dated – and preferably witnessed – notes of every discussion are essential.

Genograms (family trees)

The genogram is a quick and useful way of recording the details of the patient and their family details.

By using an agreed system of symbols, as in the genogram shown below, the patient can be quickly identified. Any other members of the family who coincidentally are also cancer sufferers can be marked as well, and this may help to identify those cases where there is a genetic link or other identifiable risk factor.

The commonly used system is shown here. Some people prefer to mark the patient by putting a cross through the relevant square or circle, and to indicate a deceased relative by filling in the circle or square, thus blacking it out.

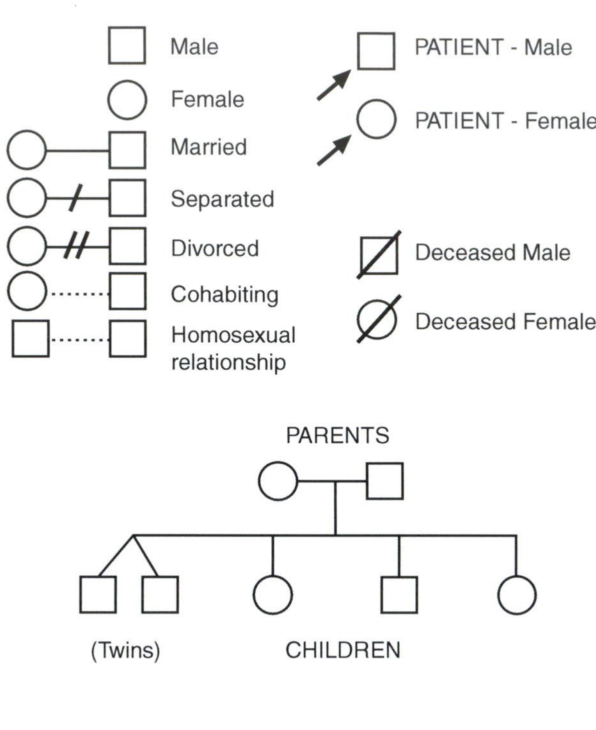

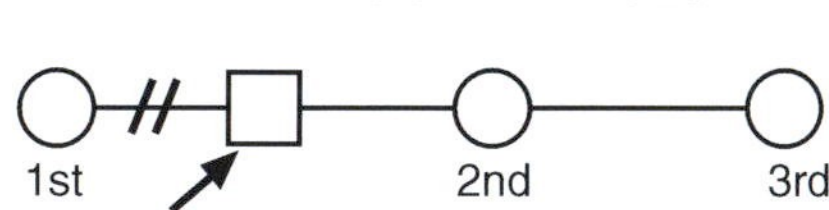

How good is that new drug?

One of the problems we all face is how to cope with the myriad new treatments that are constantly appearing on the market. Clever advertising and excellent presentation skills leave us feeling that we must at least try every new product that comes on the market. In palliative care we also face the situation where sometimes there is no evidence and one is dependent on anecdotal reports from respected and experienced colleagues where drugs are being used outwith their licence (e.g. cimetidine for malignant sweating). What can we do to help us to assess the quality and accuracy of information offered about new products? We can use the word PHARMACIST to remind us of a number of points that are worth considering.

- **P**lausible, or pharmacological explanation of the mode of action?
- **H**anging comparisons – 'It's better than drug X'. But how good is drug X?
- **A**dverse events – were they fully reported?
- **R**eproducible responses – were they seen in all of the clinical trials?
- **M**aximising the positive message – ignoring or minimising the side-effects?
- **A**dding pilot studies to randomised controlled trials?
- **C**ost or cost-effectiveness being discussed?
- **I**nverting the hierarchy of evidence with positive but unimportant messages?
- **S**tarter packs may be useful to have, but they also encourage prescribing!
- **T**rials comparing the product with placebo alone are misleading.

When deciding whether to use a new therapy, one must consider the effect of the treatment, the acceptability of the treatment to the patient, and its cost and cost-effectiveness. These may be summarised in the following grid.

Outcome	*Increased cost*	*Same cost*	*Lower cost*
Better outcome	Consider: may be justified	Accept	Accept
Same outcome	Reject	Why change?	Accept
Worse outcome	Reject	Reject	Reject

Keeping good-quality clinical records

- All pages must be clearly marked with the patient's name and reference number, preferably in the same place on each page so that omissions are easily identified.
- Allergies, blood group and other significant information should be in a different colour (e.g. red) or highlighted.
- Blank pages must be crossed out to prevent notes or amendments being added later.
- Case discussions with more than one person present require the names of all staff members who are present to be recorded.
- Drug names should always be approved pharmaceutical names or rINNs, never trade names.
- Every consultation should be recorded, dated and signed.
- Facts and opinions or clinical judgements are not the same thing, and must be kept separate. Both must be clearly identifiable.
- Notes must be sufficiently detailed, and each separate entry should refer to events that take place at one time. The person who is reading your notes should be able to know exactly what happened.
- Sign and date all entries, stating your name, grade and contact details if giving an invited opinion.
- Telephone conversations must be recorded. Who was spoken to? When? How long for? What was said?
- Use your judgement about how to record sensitive information without losing the meaning of what it says.
- Write legibly!

Do not

- Postpone making notes until later. You might forget something or record it inaccurately.
- Use non-standard abbreviations or ones that have more than one interpretation.
- Use flippant language. Patients are allowed to read their notes.
- Write anything you would not swear to under oath in a court of law.

Further reading

- Oxtoby K. Is your record keeping up to scratch? *Nurs Times.* 2004; **100:** 18–20.

Medication chart to aid compliance

This page can be photocopied for patients.

Regular medicines

Name of medication and what it is for	*Times to be taken*						
	6am	*8am*	*10am*	*12md*	*2pm*	*6pm*	*10pm*

Medications to be taken if needed

Name of medication and what it is for	*How often can I take it per 24 hours?*	*Things to report to the doctor or nurse*

Mistakes and learning from them

We all make mistakes. It is natural and normal, but we can learn from them and move on to do better in future.

If a mistake has occurred, adopt a step-by-step approach and analyse what went wrong, with determination to learn from it and not to repeat the incident.

There are five basic things to be addressed.

- The event.
- How you reacted.
- Identifying the negative points.
- Identifying the positive points.
- Moving on.

The event

- Identify what happened.
- Identify your position in relation to and responsibility for the incident.
- Identify the roles and responsibilities of others involved.
- Seek their opinion about their involvement.

How you reacted

- Accurately and honestly analyse and appraise your own actions and how they led to the mistake that occurred.
- Ask yourself when you were aware that you had made a mistake.
- Analyse your initial and subsequent actions and responses.
- Could this event have been prevented? If so, how?
- Learn how to avoid repeating the mistake, and make an appropriate action plan.

Identifying the negative points

- Identify at what point and for what reason your performance fell below the acceptable and required standard.
- Was there a genuine critical event that precipitated the mistake? Record this event.
- Look at the wider issues of team or organisational weaknesses that led to or may have contributed to the event. Do not apportion blame unfairly!

Identifying the positive points

- Are there any positive outcomes? Can there be positive outcomes? If so, start working on them now.
- Did the team support you or are there lessons that can be learned about team building for future use?

Moving on

- Consider all the learning points and share these.
- Identify and implement any improvements that are needed.
- Take appropriate steps to ensure that this event can't happen again, if possible.
- Develop new strategies to identify, develop and implement any new ways to improve the services that you and your team offer to patients.

Patients using the Internet as a source of information

There is no question that the Internet, with its much more regular updates, is leaving paper resources, with the possible exception of journals, obsolete as an up-to-date resource for obtaining recent information. This is good for professionals who have the skills necessary to recognise a reliable Internet site and to use it. However, a number of questions need to be asked about patients using the Internet.

The Hungarian psychoanalyst Michael Balint stressed that doctors must listen to their patients and that, when prescribing, the strongest drug available was in fact the doctor. Fifty years on, the tendency is to prescribe the drug that the patient will actually take, and we are much more open about side-effects and risks. Patients are much more aware and educated, and they have frequently researched the available treatments on the Internet before consulting their doctor.

This raises an important question. Is the patient sufficiently 'information literate' to accurately interpret what they find? In one survey by Schmidt, which looked at complementary medicine, the following results were obtained:[1]

- 65% of site users felt that the accuracy of the online information needed improvement
- 65% thought that the quality of information which was offered needed to be improved
- 50% had difficulty deciding what was credible and what was not trustworthy.

Schmidt suggests 10 questions that are worth asking about Internet sites.

1. Who is responsible for the website content?
2. Does the site have an editorial board?
3. Is information peer-reviewed before being posted?
4. Are the claims that are made 'too good to be true'?
5. Is information presented in scientific-sounding but obscure language?
6. Does the site promise quick, dramatic and miraculous results from the therapies described?
7. Is the author of the information on the website named? Is that person the author of the website generally, the author of the original research, or what?
8. How up to date is the information?
9. Who is paying for the maintenance of the website?
10. Is there any privacy policy?

Reference

1 Schmidt K. The World Wide Web as a medical information source for Internet users – benefits and boundaries. *Focus Altern Compl Ther.* 2004; **9:** 187–9.

Post-mortem examinations

It is never easy speaking to bereaved relatives about the reason for a post-mortem examination.

In the majority of cases, the bereaved relatives are anxious about the reason for the examination. However, if they are aware of the value of the procedure this can help them during the early, difficult days of bereavement.

It helps to focus our thinking before such a discussion if we consider the people who might benefit from such a procedure.

The bereaved relatives

- The actual cause of death is established in those situations where it was previously not certain.
- The relatives can hopefully be assured that the disease could not have been discovered earlier and that nothing was missed that should have been detected at an earlier stage.
- If the disease was inherited or could be linked to a genetic cause, you will be aware of this and have an opportunity to advise who could be at risk.
- Any undiagnosed infections (e.g. tuberculosis) will be detected, and appropriate screening can be offered.
- Guilt and self-blame should be alleviated in the light of the full information that is now made available.

The medical profession

- In those cases where there was a delay in detecting the nature of the illness or where a wrong diagnosis was made, the information gained will be used to educate and inform, hopefully preventing this from happening to another patient.
- Unusual presentations of disease are recorded, and this information is used to teach doctors and alert them to the possibility of similar situations. This information is completely anonymous – individuals cannot be identified.
- The effects of treatment can be assessed and any findings made known so that, in combination with other research, treatments can be made even more effective.

Society

- Diagnoses are examined, confirmed or corrected, and doctors learn from this.
- Medical knowledge is improved and extended.
- New diseases are discovered (e.g. AIDS, CJD and Legionnaire's disease).
- Hidden infection is revealed, thereby providing the opportunity to check for cross-infection.
- Statistical information is more accurate and directs funding, research and service provision.

Further reading

- Lomas C. Gaining consent for post-mortems. *Nurs Times.* 2006; **102:** 58–9.

Quick neurological examination

This is a very quick and superficial check of neurological function, intended only as a guide to what nerves may be affected and causing symptoms. It is not intended to replace a full neurological assessment.

Cranial nerves

I	Nasal airway; sense of smell.
II	Optic nerve head; visual acuity and fields.
III, IV and VI	Eyelids; ptosis; size, shape and symmetry of pupils; diplopia and nystagmus.
V	Facial sensation; jaw jerk; eyelid reflexes.
VII	Facial movements; taste on anterior two-thirds of tongue.
VIII	Auditory acuity; positional nystagmus; auriscopic examination.
IX	Sensation in posterior third of tongue; pharynx and pharyngeal reflexes.
X	Movement of palate and posterior pharyngeal wall; palatal and pharyngeal reflexes.
XI	Sternomastoid and trapezius muscles.
XII	Movement of the tongue.

Peripheral nerves

C5	Abduction of arm.
C5/6	Raising of forearm with arms by one's side.
C6	Pronation and supination.
C6/7	Raising and lowering of hand by bending at the wrist.
C6/7/8	Adduction of arm, lowering of forearm with arms by one's side.
C7/8 and T1	Grip strength in the hand.
L2/3	Straight leg raising.
L3/4	Straightening bent leg at knee while lying down.
L4/5	Lowering raised leg, bringing toes up towards body while lying down.
L5/S1	Bending leg at knee while lying down.
S1/2	Pressing toes towards the floor, moving foot away from body.

Reading a paper: assessing the quality of what we read

One of the less commonly used definitions of the word 'ordain' is to 'enact with authority' (*Collins English Dictionary*). We can use the ORDAIN model to assess the value and authority of a research paper.

- **O**riginality of the research.
- **R**elevance to your practice.
- **D**esign of the study.
- **A**voidance of bias.
- **I**nvestigator 'blinding' so that they don't predict or skew the results.
- **N**umerical soundness (numbers and time-scale).

Recently deceased patients: a checklist

It is upsetting for bereaved relatives to receive appointments for hospital clinics weeks after a death. A few minutes of thought and planning can prevent this, and we suggest that a form like this might help. This is based on a form that WF used in general practice.

Name, address and date of birth
NHS and hospital numbers

Date, place and time of death
Certified cause of death (a)
(b)
(c)
Death certified by Dr
Referred to coroner Y/N Post-mortem Y/N
For cremation? Y/N
Cremation form part I signed by Dr
Cremation form part II signed by Dr
Undertaker
Fees paid
Second doctor paid by on (date) / /
Bereavement follow-up will be done by (name)

Details of the death to be notified to
Chiropody
Community nurses
Hospice
Hospital clinics and teams
Social services (home help, meals on wheels, etc.)
Others (specify which agencies told, when, by whom, and who took the call)

Practice clinics and records:
Age/sex register
Clinics (specify which)
Disease registers
Flu
Over 75

Remove recall appointments for:
Smear recall
Others (specify)
Any other relevant information
Completed on / / by (name)

Reviewing a randomised controlled trial

To put your systematic reviews of randomised controlled trials (RCTs) on a 'higher level', we can use the ESCALATE model that WF utilised in small group teaching.

- **E**ligibility criteria and objectives.
- **S**earch for other relevant trials.
- **C**haracteristics of each trial.
- **A**pply eligibility and exclusion criteria.
- **L**ook for other available data.
- **A**nalysis.
- **T**horough comparison with other available analyses.
- **E**xhaustive summary of findings.

RCTs in palliative care are more difficult to conduct because of the relatively short prognosis of many of the patients and the fact that although most patients are willing to participate, many are simply unfit and cannot meet the inclusion criteria.

The subject of RCTs in children with cancer is well outside the scope of this book, but it is worth mentioning a couple of points. The number of children available for inclusion in trials tends to be small because many of the conditions are less common in children. Parents and paediatricians, while fully supporting the need for trials, may prefer to opt for standard treatments rather than trial drugs.

Stress and relaxation

Working with cancer patients is very rewarding but can be demanding. It is essential that you learn to cope with the stress and also learn to relax and care for yourself.

Stress

Stress is often defined as the 'adverse reaction people have to excessive pressure or demands placed upon them.'

Stress often presents with increasing problems associated with the following:

- concentration
- decision making
- irritability
- relaxing
- sleeping.

Try to address these issues in the following three areas:

- your behaviour
- your health
- your thinking.

Behaviour

Talk about it! Speak to colleagues and friends and, if necessary, a counsellor. Many hospices have access to professional help for their staff, and this only serves to highlight the stress associated with the job.

Working with cancer patients is stressful and demanding. It can be difficult to escape from the issues that repeatedly arise, but talking to colleagues and getting support is not a sign of weakness!

Health

Restricting alcohol intake, buying healthy food and stopping smoking are all basic and obvious. Factor in time to have a few minutes in the fresh air each day if possible, and if there is a quiet place where you can relax, use it!

Think about deep breathing and relaxation exercises. They are probably being taught to your patients. Ask the person who teaches them to teach you and the other staff. There is probably someone else waiting for another person to ask for this training first!

Thinking

We all have so many rules and regulations and protocols at work, and these are essential and unavoidable. Try to keep your private and personal life as simple as possible so that you have the freedom to relax and get away from regimented routines for a while.

Relaxation

We can define our thoughts of how we 'relax' in so many ways. Do you prefer to 'be less formal', to 'chill', to 'rest' or just to 'switch off'? You need to do at least one of these!

Maximise any opportunities at work

- Coffee time is not meant to be an opportunity to read post, make phone calls and sign forms! Is this an efficient way of working?
- Lunchtime meetings are common and can be useful, but they almost always last longer than the time allocated. Try to make some free time at lunch and get away from that desk, the sandwich lunch and the pile of paperwork! Plan ahead, book a lunch with a trusted colleague and get away to a local restaurant for an hour. It helps. You will work more efficiently later.

Relaxing at home

- There are so many ways in which we could enjoy our free time, but we need to work at this. Actively seek and find a hobby or pursuit that takes your mind off work and allows you either family time or personal time, according to your needs.
- If you are working full time and running the family taxi service every evening, can you afford to employ some help with domestic work and thereby release some quality time? You probably can.

Modern lifestyles

- Hobbies and new interests are essential.
- Physical activity suits some but not others. Would it work for you? Trial membership of a suitable venue may help you to decide.
- Regular short breaks can be better than taking a month off once a year.
- The mobile phone is a wonderful device, but is it a tool or a task master? Increasingly, we allow ourselves to be available on our mobile phones at all times. The single call from a colleague, repeated by several others, adds up to a little for them but a lot for you. Restrict the use of these out-of-hours interruptions and retain some control.

Take time now

Relax regularly. Book a long weekend off here and there by forward planning, not just long-term holiday breaks that take forever to arrive and are then over before you have had time to 'switch off'.

In summary, change your behaviour, pay attention to your physical and mental health, and start thinking about having regular short meaningful breaks. These simple strategies have worked for many people.

Supporting your colleagues

We are rightly aware of the need to communicate with our patients and to care for them effectively. It is equally important that we care for and deal with our team colleagues properly.

We offer a few simple suggestions that might help you to keep your team happy.

Constructive criticism

Lead by example, and demonstrate what needs to be done rather than telling people when they have failed to achieve a desired goal.

Empathy

Disputes, disagreements and differences of opinion will inevitably arise. Try moving your position slightly and see their point of view, and invite them to do the same for you. You might not resolve the problem, but you both might see something you had missed, and hopefully you will build mutual respect.

Inclusion

Try to involve everyone. Yes, we will get on better with some than with others, but treat everyone with respect, whatever their role in the team. The tiny cog that breaks will stop the whole machine.

Individual

It sounds obvious that we should treat everyone as an individual, but how well and how often is this done? If someone lacks motivation or seems left out, find out why this is so, and draw them in as a respected and valued member of the team.

Interest

Take an appropriate amount of interest in your colleagues at work and with regard to their personal life. Build up trust as colleagues and friends. It is about setting that individual 'comfortable distance' between yourselves, getting the balance between respect for another individual's personal privacy and offering your support in all areas of their life where you are welcome.

Positive feedback

It is all too easy to be critical and corrective, but people respond far better to effective leadership and positive feedback than to driving and negative reporting when things go wrong.

And finally ...

A man once said to me 'Be nice to the other person when you are going up in the lift. You might meet him again when you are coming down'.

Teamwork and team leading

The old saying that 'Together everyone achieves more' uses the letters from the word 'team' to good effect.

Working as a team achieves results, but a team also needs to work.

Being a role model

Teams follow their leaders. Later starts, early finishes and poor standards are copied by team members if this is what they are shown by the leader.

Delegation

- Delegate tasks to the people who have the skills to carry them out effectively and efficiently.
- Do not delegate simply to ease your own workload. You'll only add to it!

Encouragement

Defend colleagues where appropriate, cultivate an attitude of loyalty, and give credit for work well done.

Enthusiasm

Your enthusiasm builds confidence among the team members and motivates them to be more active in the team as a whole.

Clear goals and objectives

Goals should be clearly defined, specific and realistic. Deadlines must be clearly defined.

Leadership strategies

The attributes that help include the following:

- action planning for achieving team outcomes
- adaptability to changes, and encouraging this approach among the team
- calculated risk taking when necessary
- conflict resolution
- creativity
- example leadership style, as it works best
- sensitivity to the needs of team members.

Listening

When making decisions, the views of others are important. Listening is an important aspect of communication. Feedback from your team feeds the views of others to you.

Support

Give praise where it is due. Let senior colleagues know about the skills of and improvements in the younger members, and provide opportunities for their personal development.

Patience

Team building takes time. It will not happen overnight.

Working 'in TANDEM' with the patient

In order to help your patient to gain the most from consultations and their treatment, we invite you to adopt the concept of working 'in TANDEM'.

The TANDEM concept is a six-point plan that can be easily used by you and your patient.

T Think

Patients have no idea what information will be asked for in a consultation. If possible, give them some ideas, inviting them to be aware of things like how symptoms started, how long they have been present and how they may be changing with time.

A Ask

Invite patients to make a list of the things they need to know now, or at a later time when they are ready to ask. This does improve their understanding of what is going on and what to expect.

N Note

Inviting patients to make a note of relevant details such as side-effects of treatment saves time and allows for a more accurate report when they are asked about such issues some time later, when their recollection will probably be less than accurate!

D Do

Offer practical advice about how to deal with day-to-day issues and activities of daily living that will help your patient to cope better with their illness or symptoms.

E Explore

With several million websites, a vast amount of inaccurate information and spurious claims about treatment easily available, your patient will benefit from your guidance about where to obtain the best information about their illness and other relevant issues.

M More information

Some patients want basic and minimal information. Others want much more but may be afraid to ask. Be aware of this, and be prepared to offer information at the level and speed appropriate to their needs.

Writing a report for the coroner

This is something that you may well never have to do in a palliative care setting, but as one lives in an increasingly litigious society, it seems reasonable to include it here.

First, remember that the role of the coroner is to investigate the cause of death, not to accuse you of malpractice. Despite this, writing a report for them is still a daunting responsibility.

There are several questions you might ask yourself.

Why are you writing the report?

Are you writing as the team doctor, or as the on-call doctor when an event or incident occurred?

What information do you need to obtain?

Obtain and copy the full notes relating to the patient. Read them in detail before you attempt to write the report. Keep these notes safe and have them to hand for reference if any questions arise later.

Read every entry by each of the team members, and familiarise yourself with the exact sequence of events.

How should the report be presented?

Start working early after the request is received. It will take longer than you think!

Be clear and chronological in your presentation. Avoid jargon if possible, but where it is essential to use medical terminology, explain exactly what you mean by your use of technical or 'medical' language.

Avoid criticism of any colleague, and do not allude to inadequacies or inefficiencies in the system of care offered.

State clearly that the report is based on events recorded in the notes by more than one individual, and also on your own recollections and memory.

Get the report checked by a senior colleague

If any of your colleagues have submitted reports to the coroner, ask to see these as a guide to how to write the report.

A senior colleague should read your report and advise whether any changes are needed.

Your defence organisation should be invited to advise you as well.

Finally, invite the NHS trust lawyers to look at your report, as they have experience in this area. If they suggest significant changes, ask yourself why this is so. Are they protecting your personal interests or those of the NHS?

Appendix

Useful contacts for cancer patients

These pages can be copied and given to patients.

It is almost impossible to keep up to date with the vast numbers of organisations that offer advice and help to patients. We have tried to select established organisations that provide the kind of advice that is usually requested.

Macmillan CancerLine keeps an updated list of organisations, and they can be contacted by telephoning 0808 808 2020.

ACT – Association for Children with Life-Threatening or Terminal Conditions and Their Families

Tel: 0117 9221 556. Office hours 9.00am–4.30pm, Monday to Friday.
Helpline: 0870 600 0301.
Website: www.act.org.uk
Services offered: helpline, information booklets.

Action Cancer (Belfast)

Tel: 028 9080 3344. Office hours 9.00am–7.00pm, Monday to Friday.
Website: www.actioncancer.org
Services offered: advocacy, complementary therapies, information booklets, support groups.

Age Concern

Age Concern Books, Units 5 and 6, Industrial Estate, Brecon, Powys LD3 8LA.
Tel: 0870 442 2120.
Booklet: *Caring for Someone Who is Dying.*

Asian Family Counselling Service

Tel: 020 8571 3933.
Services offered: bereavement counselling, counselling.

Beacon of Hope (Mid Wales)

Tel: 01970 611 957. Office hours 9.00am–4.00pm, Monday to Friday.
Website: www.thebeaconofhope.org.uk
Services offered: advocacy, helpline, information booklets, financial assistance and holidays, respite care.

Benefits Advice Line

Helpline: 0800 0184 318. Office hours 10.00am–4.00pm, Monday to Friday.
Website: www.debtadvicebureau.org.uk
Services offered: general information, helpline, information booklets.

Bristol Cancer Help Centre

Tel: 0117 9809 500. Office hours 9.30am–5.00pm, Monday to Friday.
Helpline: 0845 1232 310.
Website: www.bristolcancerhelp.org
Services offered: complementary therapies.

Cancer Backup

Tel: 020 7606 9003. Office hours 9.00am–5.30pm, Monday to Friday.
Helpline: 0808 800 1234.
Website: www.cancerbackup.org
Services offered: advocacy, helpline, information booklets, medical information. Information is available in several languages.

Cancer Black Care

Tel: 0208 961 4151. Office hours 9.00am–5.00pm, Monday to Friday.
Website: www.cancerblackcare.org
Services offered: complementary therapies, befriending and listening, financial assistance, helpline, information booklets, support groups.

Cancer Research UK

Tel: 020 7061 8355. Office hours 9.00am–5.00pm, Monday to Friday.
Website: www.cancerhelp.org.uk
Services offered: helpline, information.

Carers UK

Tel: 0207 490 8818. Office hours 9.00am–5.00pm, Monday to Friday.
Helpline: 0808 808 7777 (10.00am–12.00pm and 2.00pm–4.00pm Wednesday and Thursday).
Website: www.carersuk.org
Services offered: helpline, information.

Complementary and Alternative Medicine

The Complementary and Alternative Medicine Specialist Library.
Website: www.library.nhs.uk/cam
Services offered: provides healthcare professionals and the public with the best available evidence for complementary and alternative medicine.

Crossroads Caring for Carers

Tel: 0845 4506 555. Office hours 9.00am–5.00pm, Monday to Friday.
Helpline: 0845 4500 350.
Website: www.crossroads.org.uk
Services offered: helpline, respite care.

Cruse Bereavement Care

Tel: 0870 167 1677. Office hours 9.00am–9.00pm, Monday to Friday, and 3.00pm–5.00pm, Saturday and Sunday.
Website: www.crusebereavementcare.org.uk
Services offered: befriending and listening, general information, helpline.

Cruse Bereavement Care Scotland national office

Tel: 01738 444 178. Office hours are described as 'variable.'
Website: www.crusescotland.org.uk
Services offered: befriending and listening, general information, helpline.

Help the Aged

207–221 Pentonville Road, London, N1 9UZ.
Tel: 020 7278 1114.
Email: publications@help the aged.org.uk
Services offered: a series of booklets, including *Planning for the End of Life*, *Planning for Choice in End of Life* and *Listening to Older People*.

Macmillan Cancer Support

Tel: 020 7840 7840. Office hours 9.00am–5.30pm, Monday to Friday.
Helpline: 0808 808 2020. Available 9.00am–6.00pm, Monday to Friday.
Website: www.macmillan.org.uk
Services offered: complementary therapies, counselling, equipment loan, financial assistance, helpline, information booklets.

Macmillan CancerLine

Tel: 0808 808 2020.
Services offered: helpline offering advice for cancer patients, information booklets.

Marie Curie Cancer Care

Tel: 0207 599 7777. Office hours 9.00am–5.00pm, Monday to Friday.
Helpline: 0800 716 146.
Website: www.mariecurie.org.uk
Services offered: general information, helpline.

National Debt Helpline

Helpline: 0808 808 4000. Available 9.00am–9.00pm, Monday to Friday.
Website: www.nationaldebtline.co.uk
Services offered: helpline.

Tak Tent Cancer Support Scotland

Tel: 0141 2110 122. Office hours 10.00am–3.00pm, Monday to Friday.
Website: www.taktent.org
Services offered: befriending and listening, complementary therapies, information booklets, support groups.

Tenovus (Wales)

Tel: 02920 196 100. Office hours 9.00am–4.00pm, Monday, Tuesday, Thursday and Friday, and 9.00am–12.30pm, Wednesday.
Helpline: 0808 808 1010. Available 9.00am–4.30pm, Monday to Friday.
Website: www.tenovus.com
Services offered: advocacy, befriending and listening, financial assistance, helpline, information booklets.

Index

abdominal swelling 88–91
analgesia 90
ascites 89–91
causes 88
diuretics 90
paracentesis 90
peritoneo-venous shunts 90
acupuncture 45
nerve pain 74
addiction fears, opioids 58, 61, 67
adjuvant analgesics 59–60
adverse drug reactions (ADRs) 41–2
agitation *see* terminal agitation/restlessness
agreement, confidentiality 27
alcohol withdrawal, confusion 113
Alexander technique 46
alfentanil, syringe drivers 80
allergy, itch 158
alternative therapies *see* complementary therapies
ambiguity, communication 3
anaemia 139
analgesia
see also pain
adjuvant analgesics 59–60
analgesic ladder, drugs 58
angry patients 19–22
anger/aggression management 270
causes 270
dos/don'ts 20–1, 270
formal complaints 21
reasons 19, 21–2
warning signs 270
anorexia 92–8
drugs 95
antagonists, drugs 39–40
antibiotics
cough 122
diarrhoea 132
sweating 194
anticonvulsants, nerve pain 74
antihistamines
itch 160
nausea/vomiting 173
aphthous ulcers, mouth problems 169
appetite improving 94–5, 96–7
aromatherapy 46
artificial hydration 232–6
dehydration 233–4
effects 232–3
ethics 232–6
reasons 233
religious beliefs 234–5
ascites, abdominal swelling 89–91
aspiration risk, dysphagia 134–5
autonomy, ethics 232
awareness, grieving process 229

bad news, breaking *see* breaking bad news
Baha'i faith 250–1
'BEFRIENDING' the patient 271–2
beneficence, ethics 232
benzocaine, mouth problems 169
benzodiazepines
breathlessness 105
confusion 113
twitching 202
benzydamine, mouth problems 169
bereavement 228–30
see also death
grieving process 229–30
time considerations 229–30
biochemical disorders, fatigue 140
bisphosphonates, hypercalcaemia 156–7
bites, itch 160
bone pain 60, 69–72
immediate control 70
long-term control 70
NSAIDs 69–70
orthopaedic treatment 71
palliative radiotherapy 71–2
spinal cord compression 70–1
bowel obstruction 99–102
see also constipation
causes 99
colic 100
constipation 99, 101
drugs 100–1

nasogastric tube feeding 101
signs/symptoms 99–100, 101
bowel wall oedema, dexamethasone 100
breaking bad news
communication 15–18
confidentiality 16
mistakes 16
SPIKES model 16–18
breakthrough pain 64–5
breast cancer, itch 160
breathlessness 103–7
anxiety management 107
breathing effectively 107
causes 103, 104
drugs 105–7
energy conservation 107
managing 105–7
pathophysiology 104–5
bronchodilators
breathlessness 105
cough 122
Buddhism 251–3
bulking agents, constipation 117
bupivicaine, cough 122

cachexia 108–10
causes 108
nutrition 108–10
calcitonin, hypercalcaemia 157
candidiasis, mouth problems 169, 170
cannabinoids, breathlessness 105
capsaicin, nerve pain 75
carbenoxolone, mouth problems 169
carbocysteine, cough 122
carcinoid syndrome, diarrhoea 132
cardiopulmonary resuscitation (CPR) 240–5
care centres, care location 209
care location 208–14
see also discharge planning
care centres 209
home 209–14
hospices 208–9
hospitals 208
websites 209
carers, family as *see* family as carers
case history, nutrition 93
charts, medication 285
checklist, death 291
Chinese herbal medicine 46
chiropractic 46
chlorpromazine
confusion 113
terminal agitation/restlessness 199
cholestasis, itch 158, 160
Christian Science 255–6
Christianity 248–50
cimetidine, sweating 194
clinical audit 273
clinical effectiveness 273
clinical records 284
clomethiazole, confusion 113
clonazepam, syringe drivers 80
clonidine
nerve pain 75
sweating 194
closeness, patients 33–4
codeine, cough 121
colic
bowel obstruction 100
hyoscine butylbromide 100
colitis, ulcerative 132
colleagues, supporting 295
collusion 23–5
honesty 23, 24
outcomes 23
combined drugs 67
common ground, communication 3–4
communication 1–36
ambiguity 3
angry patients 19–22
basic issues 2–5
breaking bad news 15–18
closeness 33–4
collusion 23–5
common ground 3–4
confidentiality 26–7
denial 28–30
deptutising staff 274
distancing oneself 31–2
listening 3, 6–14
non-verbal 6–14
pain 61
problems 2
question types 3
REACT (Respond Effectively As my Conscience Tells) 6–14
refusing to talk 35–6
summarising 4
time management 4
community care, home as care location 212
community nursing, home as care location 212
complaints, formal, angry patients 21
complementary therapies 43–9
acupuncture 45
Alexander technique 46

aromatherapy 46
Chinese herbal medicine 46
chiropractic 46
crystal therapy 47
herbal remedies 46, 47
homeopathy 47
massage 47
organisations 48–9
osteopathy 48
prevalence 43
reasons 44
reflexology 48
Reiki 48
resources 48–9
spiritual healing 48
websites 45–9
compliance aid, drugs 285
compression, lymphoedema 165
confidentiality 26–7
agreement 27
breaking bad news 16
legal issues 26
website 27
websites 27
Confucianism 253–4
confusion 111–14
alcohol withdrawal 113
causes 111–12
definitions 111
drugs 112–13
Wernicke's encephalopathy 113
constipation 99, 101, 115–19
see also bowel obstruction
causes 115–16
drugs 117–18
laxatives 117–18
opioids 117
contacts, for cancer patients 300–2
continuous subcutaneous infusion (CSCI) 78–85
cordotomy, nerve pain 75
coroner, reports for 298
corticosteroids, breathlessness 105–6
cough 120–5
causes 120–1
drugs 121–3
dry 121–2
productive 122–3
CPR *see* cardiopulmonary resuscitation
Crohn's disease, diarrhoea 132
crystal therapy 47
CSCI *see* continuous subcutaneous infusion
cyclizine, syringe drivers 80
day care units, home as care location 212, 217
death 220–7
see also euthanasia
after 224–7
bereavement 228–30
checklist 291
continuity of care 221–7
dying 220–3
end-of-life care planning 220–1
end-of-life decisions 280–1
post-mortem examinations 288
reports for coroner 298
speaking to relatives 224–7
What to Do After a Death 226
death certificate 275
definitions
confusion 111
pain 52
dehydration *see* artificial hydration
delirium, defining 111
denial 28–30
healthy/unhealthy 28–30
types 28–9
dependence fears *see* addiction fears
depression 126–30
diagnosing 126–7
drugs 128–9
fatigue 140
grieving process 229
non-pharmacological management 127–8
deputising staff, communication 274
dexamethasone
bowel wall oedema 100
spinal cord compression 190
syringe drivers 80
diamorphine
cough 122
syringe drivers 80
diarrhoea 131–3
causes 131
drugs 132–3
spurious 131
diclofenac, syringe drivers 81
dictating letters 276–7
diethylstilboestrol, sweating 194
dihydrocodeine, syringe drivers 81
dilatation, dysphagia 135
diltiazem, sweating 194
disbelief, shocked, grieving process 229
disc disease, spinal cord compression 191
discharge planning 204–7
see also care location
drugs 204

social/family issues 205–6
success/failure 207
discharge prescriptions 278–9
distancing oneself
communication 31–2
patients 31–2
diuretics
abdominal swelling 90
breathlessness 106
do not attempt resuscitation (DNAR) 240–5
domperidone, nausea/vomiting 173
dosing, drugs 58–9
drinking, artificial hydration 232–6
drowsiness
see also fatigue
causes 180
drugs
see also named drugs; pain
actions 38–42
addiction fears 58, 61, 67
adjuvant analgesics 59–60
ADRs 41–2
analgesic ladder 58
anorexia 95
antagonists 39–40
assessing new 283
bowel obstruction 100–1
breakthrough pain 64–5
breathlessness 105–7
changes, use/governance 85
charts 285
by the clock 58
combined 67
compliance aid 285
confusion 112–13
constipation 117–18
cough 121–3
depression 128–9
diarrhoea 132–3
discharge planning 204
dosing 58–9
enzyme inhibition 40
fungating wounds 148
governance changes 85
halitosis 150–1
hiccup 152, 153–4
hypercalcaemia 156–7
individual prescription 58–9
inhibition 40
interactions 41–2
lymphoedema 165
medication charts 285
mixing drugs 83–4
by mouth 58
mouth problems 169–70
nausea/vomiting 101, 173–6
nerve pain 74–7
new, assessing 283
nightmares 178–9
NSAIDs 69–70, 75
opioids 58–9, 64–7
receptors 38–9
sleep disorders 186–7
SSRIs, depression 128
sweating 194–5
syringe drivers 80–4
tenesmus 196–7
terminal agitation/restlessness 199
therapy 38–42
twitching 200–1
dying *see* death
dysphagia 134–7
causes 134, 136–7
dyspnoea 103
see also breathlessness
causes 106
treatment 106

eating *see* nutrition
empathy 34
end-of-life care planning 220–1
end-of-life decisions 280–1
enemas, constipation 118
enzyme inhibition, drugs 40
epidural abscess, spinal cord compression 191
epidural haematoma, spinal cord compression 191
epidural injections, nerve pain 76
ethics
artificial hydration 232–6
autonomy 232
beneficence 232
defining 232
euthanasia 241–3
justice 232
non-maleficence 232
principles 232
refusing treatment 237–9
resuscitation 240–5
withdrawing/withholding treatment 232–6
euthanasia 241–3
Christian Science 256
Confucianism 254
Taoism 255

faecal impaction, diarrhoea 132
faecal softeners, constipation 118
family as carers 215–19
  see also home as care location
  nursing help 216
  planning 215–19
  stress 216–17
  websites 218
family/social issues
  discharge planning 205–6
  home as care location 209–14
family trees 282
fatigue 138–41
  see also drowsiness
  anaemia 139
  causes 138–9
  defining 138
  depression 140
  nutrition 140
  sleep 140
fears, opioids 58, 61, 67–8
fentanyl
  pain 66
  syringe drivers 81
financial support
  home as care location 213
  websites 213
fistulae 142–4
Folk religions 255
food/feeding *see* nutrition
formal complaints, angry patients 21
fungating wounds 145–8

gabapentin, nerve pain 75
General Medical Council, website 27
genograms (family trees) 282
glycopyrronium, syringe drivers 81
governance changes, drugs 85
granisetron, nausea/vomiting 173
grieving process
  bereavement 229–30
  time considerations 229–30

haemoptysis 123–5
  causes 123
  massive 124
halitosis 149–51
  see also mouth problems
  causes 149–50
  drugs 150–1
hallucinations 177
haloperidol
  confusion 113
  nausea/vomiting 173
  nightmares 178
  syringe drivers 81
hearing, non-verbal communication/
    listening 8–9
herbal remedies 46, 47
hiccup 152–4
  causes 152
  drugs 152, 153–4
Hinduism 256–8
histamine release, itch 158
home as care location 209–14
  see also family as carers
  community care 212
  community nursing 212
  day care units 212, 217
  family/social issues 209–14
  financial support 213
  meals-on-wheels 213
  nursing help 212, 213
  stress 216–17
  websites 213, 218
homeopathy 47
honesty, collusion 23, 24
hospices, care location 208–9
hospitals, care location 208
Humanism 258–60
hydration, artificial *see* artificial hydration
hydromorphone
  pain 66
  syringe drivers 81
hyoscine butylbromide
  colic 100
  syringe drivers 81
hyoscine hydrobromide
  nausea/vomiting 173
  syringe drivers 82
hypercalcaemia 155–7
  causes 157
  defining 155
  drugs 156–7
  pathophysiology 156–7
  symptoms 155–6

ileal resection, diarrhoea 132
illusions 177
information source, Internet 287
inhibition, drugs 40
interactions, drugs 41–2
Internet
  see also websites
  patients' information source 287
intestinal disease, diarrhoea 132

intrathecal injections, nerve pain 76
intubation
  dysphagia 135–6
  nasogastric tube feeding 95–6
  PEG 95–6
Islam 260–2
itch 158–60
  causes 158–9

jaundice 161–2
Jehovah's Witnesses 263
Judaism 264–6
justice, ethics 232

ketamine
  nerve pain 75
  syringe drivers 82
ketorolac, syringe drivers 82

laser, dysphagia 136
laxatives
  constipation 117–18
  diarrhoea 132
leading, team 296
learning
  listening 6
  from mistakes 286
legal issues, confidentiality 26
letters, dictating 276–7
levomepromazine
  confusion 113
  nausea/vomiting 173
  syringe drivers 82
  terminal agitation/restlessness 199
listening
  communication 3, 6–14
  learning 6
  non-verbal communication 6–14
  REACT (Respond Effectively As my Conscience Tells) 6–14
liver cholestasis, itch 158, 160
location, care *see* care location
lying *see* denial
lymphoedema 163–6
  compression 165
  drugs 165
  massage 165
  pathophysiology 163–4
  signs/symptoms 164
  skin care 165–6
lymphoma, itch 160

Macmillan nurses 213, 216
malabsorption, diarrhoea 132
massage 47
  lymphoedema 165
meals-on-wheels, home as care location 213
medication charts 285
metabolic disorders, fatigue 140
methadone
  nerve pain 75
  pain 66–7
  syringe drivers 82
metoclopramide
  nausea/vomiting 173
  syringe drivers 82
metronidazole
  fungating wounds 147
  halitosis 150–1
midazolam
  cost 199
  syringe drivers 82
  terminal agitation/restlessness 199
mistakes, learning from 286
Mormonism 266
morphine
  see also opioids
  syringe drivers 82
mouth problems 167–70
  see also halitosis
  causes 167–8
  drugs 169–70
mucositis, mouth problems 170
myoclonic jerks 200–1
myths
  opioids 67–8, 180, 238–9
  syringe drivers 78

naproxen, sweating 194
nasogastric tube feeding 95–6
  bowel obstruction 101
nausea/vomiting 171–6
  causes 171–2, 174–6
  drugs 101, 173–6
  non-pharmacological management 172
neoplastic fever, sweating 194
nerve blocks
  nerve pain 75
  tenesmus 197
nerve pain 73–7
  acupuncture 74
  causes 73
  cordotomy 75
  drugs 74–7
  nerve blocks 75
  neurolytic procedures 75

radiotherapy 76
spinal injections 76
TENS (transcutaneous electrical nerve stimulation) 76
neurological examination 289
neurolytic procedures, nerve pain 75
news, bad *see* breaking bad news
night terrors 178
nightmares 177–9
defining 177
drugs 178–9
opioids 178
non-maleficence, ethics 232
non-pharmacological management
depression 127–8
nausea/vomiting 172
sleep disorders 187
sweating 194
terminal agitation/restlessness 198–9
non-verbal communication/listening 6–14
hearing 8–9
sight 7–8
smell 9–10
taste 10–11
touch 11–12
NSAIDs
bone pain 69–70
nerve pain 75
nursing help
family as carers 216
home as care location 212, 213
Macmillan nurses 213, 216
nutrition
anorexia 92–8
appetite improving 94–5, 96–7
assessment 93–4
cachexia 108–10
case history 93
fatigue 140
nasogastric tube feeding 95–6
PEG 95–6
taste 10–11, 97

octreotide, syringe drivers 83
odour
fungating wounds 147
halitosis 149–51
oesophageal thrush, dysphagia 134
ondansetron
nausea/vomiting 173
syringe drivers 83
opioid-induced itch 160
opioid-induced sedation 180–1
opioids
addiction fears 58, 61, 67
alternatives 65–7
breathlessness 106
constipation 117
diarrhoea 133
fears 58, 61, 67–8
fentanyl 66
hydromorphone 66
methadone 66–7
myoclonic jerks 201
myths 67–8, 180, 238–9
nerve pain 76
opioid-resistant pain 65
opioid-responsive pain 66
oxycodone 66
pain 58–9, 64–7
refusing treatment 238–9
osmotic agents, constipation 118
osteopathy 48
oxycodone, pain 66
oxygen, breathlessness 106

pain 51–85
see also drugs
adjuvant analgesics 59–60
assessment 53–6
bone pain 60, 69–72
breakthrough pain 64–5
causes 53, 65
communication 61
components 53
definitions 52
describing 54–6
fungating wounds 147
managing 57–62
mouth 169
nerve pain 73–7
opioid-resistant 65
opioid-responsive 65
opioids 58–9, 64–7
out of control 63–8
persistent 63–8
PQRSTUV principles 54
scales 54–6
spinal cord compression 188–90
syringe drivers 78–85
terminology 52
treatment options 57–62
palliative radiotherapy, bone pain 71–2
papers, reading 290
paracentesis, abdominal swelling 90
paraneoplastic syndrome, itch 160

patients
  closeness 33–4
  distancing oneself 31–2
  empathy 34
  Internet, information source 287
  websites 300–2
percutaneous endoscopic gastrostomy (PEG) tube feeding 95–6
peritoneo-venous shunts, abdominal swelling 90
persistent pain 63–8
phenobarbital
  syringe drivers 83
  terminal agitation/restlessness 199
pholcodine, cough 122
planning
  discharge 204–7
  end-of-life care 220–1
  family as carers 215–19
plicamycin, hypercalcaemia 157
post-mortem examinations 288
post-radiation xerostomia, mouth problems 170
PQRSTUV principles, pain assessment 54
prescriptions, discharge 278–9
pressure ulcers 182–5
  causes 182–3
  educating the family 185
  pathogenesis 182–3
  prevention 183–4
  treatment 184
  websites 185
prochlorperazine, nausea/vomiting 173
promethazine, syringe drivers 83

question types, communication 3

radiotherapy
  bone pain 71–2
  cough 123
  dysphagia 136
  nerve pain 76
  spinal cord compression 191
randomised controlled trials (RCTs), reviewing 292
ranitidine, syringe drivers 83
rashes, itch 160
RCTs *see* randomised controlled trials
REACT (Respond Effectively As my Conscience Tells), listening/communication 6–14
reading papers 290
receptors, drugs 38–9
records, clinical 284
reflexology 48
refusing treatment 237–9
Reiki 48
relaxation, stress 293–4
religious beliefs, artificial hydration 234–5
religious/spiritual issues 246–68
  Baha'i faith 250–1
  Buddhism 251–3
  Christian Science 255–6
  Christianity 248–50
  Confucianism 253–4
  Folk religions 255
  Hinduism 256–8
  Humanism 258–60
  Islam 260–2
  Jehovah's Witnesses 263
  Judaism 264–6
  Mormonism 266
  Sikhism 267–8
  Taoism 254–5
renal failure, itch 160
reports, for coroner 298
resolution, grieving process 229–30
resources
  see also websites
  complementary therapies 48–9
restlessness *see* terminal agitation/restlessness
resuscitation 240–5
  CPR 240–5
  DNAR 240–5
risperidone, confusion 113

sadness 126–30
saline
  breathlessness 106
  cough 122
sedation, opioid-induced 180–1
sex hormone insufficiency, sweating 194
shocked disbelief, grieving process 229
sight, non-verbal communication/listening 7–8
Sikhism 267–8
skin care, lymphoedema 165–6
skin ulceration risk *see* pressure ulcers
sleep disorders 186–7
  drugs 186–7
  nightmares 177–9
  non-pharmacological management 187
sleep, fatigue 140
smell, non-verbal communication/listening 9–10

social/family issues
discharge planning 205–6
home as care location 209–14
SPIKES model, breaking bad news 16–18
spinal cord compression 70–1, 188–92
chemotherapy 190
disc disease 191
epidural abscess 191
epidural haematoma 191
pain 188–90
progression 188–9
radiotherapy 191
signs/symptoms 188, 189–90
steroids 191
surgery 191
spinal injections, nerve pain 76
spiritual healing 48
spiritual/religious issues 246–68
defining spirituality 246
SSRIs, depression 128
St John's Wort, depression 129
steatorrhea, diarrhoea 132
steroids
dysphagia 136
hypercalcaemia 157
nausea/vomiting 173–4
nerve pain 76
spinal cord compression 191
sweating 194
stimulants, constipation 118
stress 293–4
family as carers 216–17
home as care location 216–17
relaxation 293–4
sucralfate, mucositis 170
summarising, communication 4
supporting colleagues 295
suppositories, constipation 118
surgery, spinal cord compression 191
sweating 193–5
causes 193, 195
drugs 194–5
infection 194
neoplastic fever 194
non-pharmacological management 194
sex hormone insufficiency 194
syringe drivers 78–85
discontinuing CSCI 84–5
drugs 80–4
indications 79
mixing drugs 83–4
myths 78
websites 85

'in TANDEM', working with the patient 297
Taoism 254–5
taste
altered 10, 97
non-verbal communication/ listening 10–11
nutrition 10–11
team leading 296
teamwork 296
tenesmus 196–7
drugs 196–7
nerve blocks 197
TENS (transcutaneous electrical nerve stimulation), nerve pain 76
terminal agitation/restlessness 198–9
defining 111
drugs 199
non-pharmacological management 198–9
theophyllines, breathlessness 106
therapies 38–49
alternative 43–9
complementary 43–9
drugs 38–42
tics 201
time considerations, grieving process 229–30
time management, communication 4
tiredness *see* drowsiness; fatigue
touch, non-verbal communication/ listening 11–12
tramodol, syringe drivers 83
treatment
refusing 237–9
withdrawing/withholding 232–6
tremors 201
tricyclic antidepressants
depression 128
nerve pain 76–7
twitching 200–2
benzodiazepines 202
causes 200–1
drugs 200–1
myoclonic jerks 200–1
tics 201
tremors 201

ulceration, skin *see* pressure ulcers
ulcerative colitis, diarrhoea 132

vomiting *see* nausea/vomiting

weakness *see* fatigue
websites
  for cancer patients 300–2
  care location 209
  complementary therapies 45–9
  confidentiality 27
  family as carers 218
  financial support 213
  General Medical Council 27
  home as care location 213, 218
  for patients 300–2
  pressure ulcers 185
  syringe drivers 85
Wernicke's encephalopathy, confusion 113
withdrawing/withholding treatment 232–6
working 'in TANDEM' with the patient 297
wounds, fungating 145–8

zoledronic acid, hypercalcaemia 157